LET THE RIVERSIDE MOTHERS GROUP SHOW YOU . . .

➤ How to make your baby's room a comfortable, imaginative play area—simple, inexpensive tips

➤ Diaper diversions—how to keep changing from being a battle

➤ Social pleasures—the best ways to introduce your baby to other babies

➤ Alternatives to "no"—making the "N word" meaningful

➤ Shopping tips to save time, money, and aggravation

➤ How to pick a baby-friendly vacation spot

➤ How to create an island of peace for yourself

It's all here, and much more in.

ENTERTAIN ME!

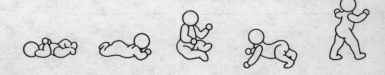

ENTERTAIN ME!

Creative Ideas for Fun and Games with Your Baby in the First Year

The Riverside Mothers Group

POCKET BOOKS

New York   London   Toronto   Sydney   Tokyo   Singapore

Parental supervision and discretion are advised when following the advice and suggestions in this book. The authors and publisher disclaim any liability arising directly or indirectly from the use of this book.

An *Original* Publication of POCKET BOOKS

POCKET BOOKS, a division of Simon & Schuster Inc.
1230 Avenue of the Americas, New York, NY 10020

Copyright © 1993 by The Riverside Mothers Group
Illustrations by Sharon D. Siegel, copyright © 1993

DESIGN: Stanley S. Drate/Folio Graphics Co. Inc.

Library of Congress Cataloging-in-Publication Data

Entertain me! / the Riverside Mothers Group.
    p.   cm.
  Includes bibliographical references.
  ISBN 0-671-74536-0
  1. Play—Miscellanea. 2. Creative activities and seatwork—
Miscellanea. 3. Infants—Care—Miscellanea. I. Riverside
Mothers Group.
HQ782.E55   1993
649'.51—dc20   93-6983
                                                 CIP

First Pocket Books trade paperback printing July 1993

10 9 8 7 6 5 4 3 2

Printed in the U.S.A.

To our children:

Anna Regine Campbell
Molly Ruth Campbell
George Abraham Siegel Duffy
William Scott Siegel Duffy
Kara Rebecca Kellam Fowler
Anna Sophia Nachamie
Samuel McKenzie Newman
Eliza Paige Newman
Jenny Persons Vallancourt
Sarah Persons Vallancourt

and to new parents and babies everywhere

Our deepest gratitude to Claire Zion (and her daughter, Rose), Angela Kyle, Jane Ginsberg and Michael Sanders at Pocket Books. Our heartfelt thanks to Robin Rue (and her daughter, Rosina) and the good folks at the Anita Diamant Literary Agency.

Our warmest appreciation to those who helped and inspired us: Sharon D. Siegel, our wonderful illustrator; Fretta Reitzes, Beth Teitelman, the entire staff and all the babies, mothers, and caregivers at the 92nd Street "Y" Parenting Center; Diane McNamara and the entire staff at the West Side YMCA children's programs; Arlene Eisenberg; Penelope Leach; Sandee Brawarsky; Chuck Newman; David Vallancourt; Howard Nachamie; Ben Fowler; Ed Campbell; Bob Campbell; Chris Hunt; Janet Krober; Michelle Brauntuch; Cindy Solomon; Jeannie and Arthur Sammeth; Patricia Goldstein; Earlene Williams; Herminia Resto; Tracy Warwick; Kenlyn Kirby; Anya Bernstein; Li Li and Zhen Li Li.

Thanks also to the helpful people at the New York Public Library, Eeyore's Books for Children, the Bank Street College Book Store, and West Side Kids.

Note to Readers

We used the pronouns "he" and "she" in alternate chapters when referring to the generic baby. The introduction is he, "Basic Training," she, and so forth.

A Guide to the Players

Hedy and Ed Campbell are the parents of Molly.

Laurie Sammeth Campbell and Bob Campbell are the parents of Anna.

Genny Kellam and Ben Fowler are the parents of Kara.

Libby Mark and Chuck Newman are the parents of Sam and Eliza.

Lois and Howard Nachamie are the parents of Annie (Blazer is their dog).

Jil Persons and David Vallancourt are the parents of Jenny.

Paula Siegel and Steven Duffy are the parents of George and Will.

Contents

PART
III
_____

Appendices

Introduction

Congratulations on your new baby. How wonderful! And how exhausting and overwhelming.

For most parents, having a baby is a huge change that leaves many initially racked with self-doubt and is only worsened by the debilitating effects of too little sleep. Then there are the endless niggling yet important decisions that go hand in hand with baby care. Is it too soon to feed the baby again? Is one sweater enough when we go out today? Are there enough blankets on the crib?

Take heart. Newborns' lives are full of predictable (albeit shifting) cycles. They eat, they burp, they make good use of their diapers, they sleep. The highlight is when a newborn sleeps: you get to eat, shower, nap, and read this book. You'll discover your baby's patterns soon enough.

Babies also cry. It's natural. Sometimes they cry simply because they're hungry, wet, or tired. But sometimes it's harder to figure out the cause of the baby's distress. Look at that face. Why is it crumpling? It may be boredom. Could the baby be asking to play?

Play? Play how? With what? Your baby can't even sit up yet? No problem.

A baby is never too young to begin playing. Your first games will calm and comfort your newborn. Later you'll use play to distract, divert, and entertain him. Games, especially those meant to be played while you wend your way through nonstop baby-care tasks, will make life much more pleasant for you both. Simply put, play is baby magic. It stimulates and reassures. It works.

Experts will tell you that play heightens babies' interest in what's going on around them, helps them learn how to focus and concentrate on a task, and aids the development of their coordination and dexterity. By playing with their parents, relatives, and sitters, babies learn fundamental social skills of communication and cooperation. Later, playing by themselves will encourage self-reliance and help them learn to make decisions and to pick the right tool for the right job. Big stuff for ones so little.

As mothers, we know that having fun with a baby makes the difference between an endless, tedious, custodial sort of day and one punctuated with a smile here, a chuckle there. Playing is how we learned about our babies' personalities, preferences, abilities, and limits.

Please don't get the idea that all seven of us sailed through every waking second of every day of our babies' first years. If those twelve months had been a breeze, the Riverside Mothers Group (named after our local oasis, Riverside Park) would never have been formed and this book would never have been written (see Chapter 9, "Peer Pleasure," for the nuts and bolts of forming a play group).

What we learned from firsthand experience, one another, and the benefits of hindsight we share with you in this book. We also gratefully acknowledge our husbands, sitters, families, pediatricians, and countless strangers who offered their unsolicited advice. Seven moms created this book, so the ideas and suggestions reflect our combined experiences with nine very different kids.

We've met weekly since our babies were around six months old to share confidences, advice, worries, solutions, and pride (the kids are now all past four). In the course of our collective first year, the mysteries of new parenthood faded and our sense of competency strengthened. We discovered that we knew more than we thought we did. You will, too.

How to Use This Book

Entertain Me! is a collection of games, rhymes, songs, tips, tricks, ideas, and advice to see new parents through this topsy-turvy but exhilarating first year. The first of the book's three parts, "Getting Through the Day," shows you how to introduce play during the initial settling-in period with a newborn and as you go about taking care of the baby's needs. In Part II, "Let the

Games Begin," we get into games, toys, music, books, travel, and play groups, all of which add to the fun. Appendices in Part III include song lyrics, mail-order sources, and tips for the first birthday. We hope you will use the book as a resource and as a springboard for your own inventions.

We balked at books that affixed signs of developmental progress to specific ages. Worrying that your baby is slower or faster than the "norm" just feeds insecurities and adds to sleep loss. Egad, what if your darling is merely average? Our kids all rolled over, cut teeth, talked, walked, and picked up raisins between thumb and forefinger at different ages.

However, while writing this book we found it useful to attribute some age ranges to certain games: they are meant as approximations—ballpark-sized approximations—of when _your baby_ may begin to enjoy a certain game, toy, song, or whatever.

We've divided the first year into five loosely defined, overlapping developmental categories. The corresponding symbols, which appear in the margins throughout the book, will help you spot the text for your baby's age group.

Newborns are babies who haven't yet really woken up to the world (0–2 months).

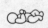**Lap babies** are the ones who are alert and can support their heads but cannot yet sit up (2–7 months).

Sitters, obviously, can sit up by themselves without slumping over like boneless chickens (4–9 months).

Crawlers are babies who have discovered mobility, either by creeping or crawling (6–11 months).

Cruisers are the terrors who can pull themselves upright and navigate around anything as long as they have something to hold on to (7 months and up).

Heart symbol means appropriate for, or applicable to, all babies during the first year.

Because relatively few babies walk unassisted before their first birthdays, we have not included a separate category for walkers. The advice in the cruisers' sections will serve parents of pre-one walkers well.

Games geared toward crawlers and cruisers may seem more plentiful and more fun, but that's because your baby's abilities will blossom in the second half of his first year. Many of the games age well. Some you'll start using in his infancy and never give up. Others you'll modify as your baby grows.

Remember, what your child wants more than any toy in the world only you can provide. Your love, affection, and attention are the best gifts of all. You are the ideal parent for your little one because you are doing your best to respond to your baby's needs with flexibility, imagination, and skill. And you're getting better at it every day. Respect yourself for doing the most difficult job in the world. Go with your instincts. Do what pleases you both. The key is to have fun because, as Dr. Seuss wrote, "Fun is good."

PART

I

Getting Through the Day

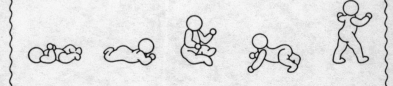

1

BASIC TRAINING

Soothing, Changing, Dressing, and Bathing

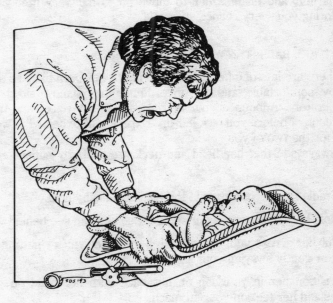

In the first weeks, the baby's entertainment won't be your top priority. After all, a newborn isn't the most playful creature in the world. Nonetheless, you can ease her into her first games as you tend to her waking needs.

Pat the soles of her feet together as you change her. Blow on her bare tummy as you dress her. Kiss her knees while you give her a sponge bath. Add a nonsense phrase or song. Every time you play one of these little games, you teach her a tiny bit more about life, get her more accustomed to the rituals of babyhood, and help her feel safe and happy.

Soothing

You start to play with your baby simply and naturally the moment you take her in your arms. As you hold her, she grows accustomed to your face, touch, smell. As you talk to her—as if she understands every word you say from her first days—she'll come to recognize that your voice and presence mean comfort. Chatting about what you see and do together is the hands-down first, best, and most portable game during the first year. This soothes her, calms her, and enables her to move on to her very first game: exploring you every chance she gets.

I GOT YOU, BABE: TEN WAYS TO HOLD A BABY

There are lots of different ways to hold a newborn baby so she's happy, comfortable, and receptive. Remember to move slowly and deliberately. Announce your arrival with a soft voice, and make eye contact before you pick her up. Experiment to see what works well for the two of you.

Always see that her head and neck are properly supported as you

➤ Cradle her in your arms in the traditional baby hold.

➤ Hold her snugly over your shoulder so she can see behind you.

➤ Put her across your knees with her face down; try patting her back or gently swaying your legs.

➤ Position her in your lap on her back with her head on your knees and her feet on your stomach.

➤ Prop her up in your lap looking out.

➤ Carry her like a football: cup the back of her head in your hand, position her body along your arm, and tuck her against your side.

➤ Use the "fire fighter hold," her ear cupped in your hand, her tummy along your forearm, and her back tucked against your side.

➤ "Seat" her propped in the crook of your arm, her back against your chest, while you walk around.

➤ Lay her prone on your stomach while you lie down.

➤ Strap her into an infant carrier—few things are as comforting to your baby as her little head against your heart—as you go about your day.

Bear in mind that while some babies love being held morning till night, some get cranky when handled too much. They get "overstimulated" with attention and end up fussing. From her earliest days, your baby will let you know what she prefers by her body language. If she pulls away or averts her eyes, it may be a signal to stop the excitement and let her catch her breath.

Similarly, let sleeping (and happy) babies lie. If the baby is not crying, don't feel compelled to present her with a sideshow. Some babies are perfectly content to spend lots of time watching the world go by with occasional attention from you. Thank your lucky stars and indulge yourself in those "gift moments."

ROCK-A-BYE BABY

Gentle motion, for most newborns (and older babies too), is nirvana; in fact, it's wonderfully soothing for both of you. With newborns, keep the rocking slow and easy. You can hold her while you sway from side to side, back and forth, or rock her up and down in your arms. Get cozy in a rocking chair and rock while humming and patting her rhythmically on her back or bottom.

Other ways to use movement with a small baby (accompanied by background music, if you like), many of which are wonderful calming techniques with cranky or colicky babies, are

➤ Walk, sway, or slow-dance with the baby on your shoulder (try different holds).

➤ With your arms out and palms up, position the baby with her belly on your right forearm and her head looking over your left elbow. "Fly" her very gently back and forth.

➤ Hold the baby over your shoulder as you bend and straighten your knees. You can say, "Bob goes the baby. Bob goes Mom."

➤ Lie down with the baby on your chest, her ear near your comforting heartbeat.

➤ Lay the baby on your bed and bounce her very gently with a rhythmic pat on her back.

➤ Take her for a spin in the carrier or stroller or rock her in her cradle or swing.

➤ Try a porch swing or hammock (maybe you'll both get in a nap).

As you try different holds and rocking techniques on a cranky baby, don't abandon ship right away if it seems the baby is slow to calm. Give it a minute or two before you decide that what you're doing is not working. Then change the baby's position or view, or change the pace of your rocking. (Colicky babies tend to respond well to more vigorous and/or constant motion.) Try a different song, or crank up the musical mobile if you think she's tired of your voice. Massage works wonders with some fussbugets (there are several good books on infant massage; check at your local library, bookstore, or health food store).

INTO THE MOUTHS OF BABES

Tiny ones love to suckle; basic oral gratification is a baby's idea of fabulous fun completely apart from her need for nourishment. Each baby will express her own preferences, but they all need to suck something, sometime.

If you're breast-feeding on demand, you'll sometimes feel as if you've done nothing but nurse the baby all day. Sometimes you *will* have done nothing but nurse the baby all day. If you have the time, stamina, and inclination to gratify the baby's need to suck by nursing, your time will be well spent; you will have provided your baby with just the "entertainment" she craved.

Some babies are choosy, accepting a nipple (real or artificial) only when they want to suck and refusing pacifiers. Some will deign to use one particular brand. Others are content with anything that comes within range: any sort of pacifier, your chin, knuckle, or fingertip.

Don't be afraid of "hooking" your baby on a pacifier. Ask your pediatrician, consult the authorities, or trust us: for the first three months, if it works, use it. Later, if you want the baby to give up the pacifier, you can encourage substitutions.

As her attention span and coordination grow, her suckling will depend less and less on you. Eventually, you can help her find her own fingers and fist. By her fifth month or so, she may begin to awkwardly bring teethers and other toys to her mouth. Toward the end of the year, you can assume that she'll mouth almost anything with which she plays.

HANGING AROUND THE HOUSE

By simply carrying your little one around the house as you putter, you are giving her a wonderful opportunity to see what this Life Outside the Womb business is all about. You are also nurturing intimacy, security, and a sense of home. See how well you're doing already?

So, talk to her about this and that as you make your way through your day together. Your voice teaches, soothes, calms, reassures, and amuses her. Talk, hum, and sing as you play. Tell the baby what you are doing as you do it. ("Wow! Look at that tuna. Spoon, spoon, spoon it into the casserole. Mix, mix, mix it with the mac, mac, macaroni.") Anything that springs from your lips will work. This is no time to be self-conscious. Just keep your voice animated and translate specific emotions in your facial expressions. (A baby's visual range is only about eight to twelve inches through the first six weeks of life.) You'll find yourself babbling a lot, but that's great. The baby loves listening to you.

JIL: *David and I couldn't wait to start reading* Winnie the Pooh, *one of our favorite books, to Jenny. So when she was two weeks old, we pulled out an old copy. We knew she had no idea what we were saying, yet she enjoyed listening and we got to convey our love of Pooh.*

Yet there'll come a point, usually in mid-afternoon, when *you* think the sound of your own voice is going to shatter your sanity. In this case, you can substitute background sound, such as:

➤ any music. Some babies love reggae, others the Beatles, others classical, still others jazz; start with what *you* like and go from there.

➤ a wind chime

➤ the radio, stereo, or television

➤ a running washing machine (some babies also like the vibrations)

➤ a loudly ticking clock

➤ running or splashing water

➤ street noise

➤ a tape recording of your voice or of the baby's own gurgles, coos, and babbles

In fact, it can't hurt to keep the radio on when you are at home. You'll pick up new songs and melodies, which always come in handy as you play, and your little sponge is absorbing sound for her own amusement. Take a minute to dance together when your favorite song comes on. You may even catch a news broadcast to alleviate that "I have no idea what's going on in the world" gap most new parents experience.

Once babies can support their heads on their rubbery little necks, (anywhere from about four weeks on), they love having a good look around and seem to really enjoy variety. It's no wonder they like to be held over your shoulder: the view's great. Bear in mind that a house tour will entertain a baby of any age, anywhere, in all kinds of weather.

Newborns will focus best on patterned surfaces such as printed wallpaper, decorative tiles, grids, venetian blinds, shelved books, banisters, and railings.

Talk about what the baby's seeing and what you're doing as you make your way from room to room. At first, she'll just like the sound of your voice (even with your mouth full), no matter what you're talking about. Toward the end of the year, she'll start to absorb words and meanings and begin building her vocabulary.

As you go:

➤ Stop to show the baby her own face as you pass mirrors (see the section on mirror games, in Chapter 2, "Domestic Bliss").

➤ Introduce her to family members in the photographs on your walls.

➤ Explain what goes on in each room.

➤ Dabble her tootsies or fingers in water.

➤ Look at flowers, touch anything textural, smell dinner cooking, and listen to a light switch click, a clock chime, or the doorbell ring (and say hello to this wonderful person who brought us pizza).

➤ Turn on ceiling fans so she can watch the blades go around and around and enjoy the breeze.

JIL: _Jenny has always loved wind or a simulation of wind. In her first three months she was colicky, and one of the things that sometimes helped was to fan her. It literally took her breath away._

And don't forget to stop at windows; they're natural baby pleasers because they frame giant moving pictures. Whether you live on Broadway, Chestnut Lane, or Rural Route #2, there's always something to see out the window. Notice what time the school buses, street sweepers, or letter carriers come by, and make it a point to watch for them. Or just see what you can see: fireflies twinkling, snow falling, a neighbor working in the yard, children playing.

GENNY: _From about three months on, Kara loved staring out the window and was instantly soothed by it. (Our tenth-floor apartment overlooks a city park and the Hudson River.) As she got older, she loved finding the moon, looking for boats, picking out dogs, and pointing out fellow strollerees._

WHERE ELSE TO PLAY

There are, by the way, lots of places besides your arms or lap that are fine for playing together. In addition to wherever the spirit moves you, how about

➤ in her bassinet, cradle, or crib

➤ on a blanket or bed

➤ on the couch

➤ on her changing table

➤ on the porch, in the backyard, or at a park

New baby products and nifty gizmos are marketed each year. Most are designed as conveniences for parents, but all are fun for the baby as well. Be open-minded about locations for play and about using outside equipment (car seats, strollers, etc.) inside. If the baby enjoys watching you write thank you notes (read them aloud in a singsong voice) from her swing, great.

Sometimes, moving out of your arms or lap is just the distraction a cranky baby needs. See if the baby likes to play while

➤ in a rocking or bouncing infant seat or car seat

➤ you "wear" her in a carrier such as a Snugli or Sling

➤ in her carriage or stroller

➤ in a mechanical swing or bucket swing

➤ in a walker or jumper, a seat that hangs from stretchy cables affixed to a door frame (check with your pediatrician)

➤ in a high chair or clip-on seat

➤ in a playpen

Incidentally, if you plan to use a playpen, set it up and get her accustomed to it *before* she begins crawling. Otherwise she'll just feel confined and drag her tippy cup across the mesh side asking to see the warden. And don't crowd the playpen with too many toys. Her favorite game will be tossing them out of the playpen for you to pick up. Some parents recommend rotating playpen toys periodically so the baby won't get bored. Others think keeping certain toys strictly for playpen use works as an incentive; the baby will want to go in so she can play with them.

Activity boxes that strap onto playpens, car seat toys, stroller accessories, suction-cupped whirligigs for high chairs, and other amusements add to the fun. Plastic links (the sturdier the better) are great for connecting little toys to larger equipment.

Once the baby can sit up by herself steadily, you can take her from one room to another (if you don't have wall-to-wall carpeting) by sitting her in the middle of a bath mat or scatter rug and *slowly* pulling one end.

T I P ➤ As your baby begins to stretch, roll over, push up, and creep, expect to spend a lot of time on the floor. If your house isn't carpeted—and when you venture away from home—keep some padded quilts or mats around for both comfort and safety. (Same advice if you have wool floor coverings, which may irritate a baby's bare skin.)

Next comes mobility, an exciting development but, like all developments, one to which you'll have to adjust. It's liberating to notice that the baby's beginning to initiate games and play on her own. It's also terrifying because she's off and crawling as soon as her little knees hit the ground.

It used to be that you plunked her down and she played with whatever toys you put within her reach. Now that she can move a few inches, she will want to plot her own course. This may annoy you when you're trying to wrestle her shoes on to get to the post office before it closes. Try to be flexible. Give in to those little derailments. Sometimes just a couple of minutes under the piano stool or picking at the nubs of the welcome mat is all she'll need before she'll happily sit still.

Give the baby some playtime in which she can explore her own path. If you can leave yourself some time in which all you have to

---

T I P ➤ Babies learn early on that telephones are competition. Our advice is: when the phone rings and you're in midgame with your little one, tell the caller you'll call back. After you've gotten the baby settled with a toy, or put to bed, or in the arms of another, you call back.

When you just have to take the call, make use of the tried-and-true Telephone Fake-Out game. Hold the baby on your lap facing you. Pretend you're talking directly and exclusively to him; he doesn't know you aren't . . . yet. (Similarly, Molly's dad once lulled her to sleep by reading something he was interested in—an article about a boxing match from *Sports Illustrated.*)

---

do is follow along, so much the better. All babies dawdle and learn from their dallying. This exploration stuff is exhilarating for your baby and can be a pleasant respite for you.

Crawlers, cruisers, and walkers enjoy slightly more sophisticated household games. Try going on a treasure hunt for the cat, a favorite toy, or everything of one kind (balls, bears, or bunnies). Or let her find the source of a noise like the dishwasher or the radio you left on in another room.

Changing Time

Some babies lie back, stick their chubby legs in the air, and gurgle during diaper changes. Some cry, writhe, wriggle, and perform maneuvers that Harry Houdini would have envied. Some do both or either depending on their mood, age, the weather, their horoscope . . .

For the first diaper changes, concentrate only on the matter at hand. Handle your newborn gently, move her slowly, talk to her constantly (a running narrative on any topic will do fine), or hum a soothing tune. If the baby wails as you put her down for the change, pick her up and comfort her. Next time you lay her down, support her head and neck with one hand. Try propping her head up a bit with a folded cloth diaper or blanket. Some babies simply don't like being flat on their backs. You may have to repeat the process a few times till she gets used to it.

As you get more accustomed to the baby and the process, you can

➤ Give her a cloth diaper or other object to hold, mouth, and inspect.

➤ Install a mobile over the changing area and wind it up as you start.

➤ Tell her what you are doing every step of the way using an exaggerated voice to keep her attention on you.

➤ Tape up pictures at her eye level alongside the changing table. Talk about the pictures and, when she's old enough, ask her to look for things in the pictures.

➤ Sing any old song with as much animation and gusto as you think she can handle.

➤ Take her feet in your hands as she's lying on her back, and chant "Footsie, footsie, footsie" boogie-woogie style as you bring her feet up to remove the old diaper and "Baby, baby, baby" as you bring her feet back down. Repeat as you place the fresh diaper under her until you're done.

By the half-year mark, babies will enjoy being amused and changed at the same time. The trick is to involve them in the process, to be fast (line up everything you'll need before you start), and to make good use of distractions. Some basics:

➤ Keep a basket of little toys, preferably ones that squeak or move, by the changing table for her to hold. Rotate them often to keep the game fresh.

➤ Give her a clean diaper to inspect. Point out the little cartoon figures and patterns on the waistband of disposable diapers and talk about them.

➤ Say, "Ooo, look!" and show her something truly interesting (her hairbrush, your wristwatch, your lizard imitation, or something out the window).

➤ Wear a diaper (we suggest a clean one) on your head.

➤ Make up a silly diaper-changing ditty. Genny and Ben invented this for Kara (and Howie a similar one for Annie): "Heinie up" (lift the baby's bottom and slide the diaper under). "Heine down" (put the baby's bottom down on the diaper). "Heinie, heinie, all around" (hold the baby's thighs and make a circle in the air with them). Of course you can use fanny, tushy, bottom, whatever name you prefer for that part of your baby's body.

➤ Starting at her head, tickle each part of her body as you work your way down to her toes, stopping briefly to open the pins, Velcro, or tapes on one side on the way down. Do the other side as you work your way back up. Name the parts of the baby's body as you tickle them.

➤ Freeze and see what your baby does to reanimate you.

As your baby nears the one-year mark and gets more and more active, changing her may seem to you much like alligator wrestling. Unsnap, unbutton, and unzip her en route to the changing table. Also:

➤ Plan to do something your baby loves immediately after the diaper change and talk about it as you change her.

➤ Vary the scenery and change her diaper in a different location (on your bed, the couch, the living room floor, under the dining room table, if you have to).

➤ Invent a new "clean diaper time" song to any melody that suits you.

➤ Save a favorite picture book for her diaper changes. Prop it up by her head as you change her and turn the page now and then.

Take heart. As your baby gets older, she'll need changing less often. And one day—yes, that day will come—she won't need changing at all.

Dressed to Thrill

She won't need you to dress her forever, either. For now, though, get used to it. As for diaper changing, participation, distractions, games, and songs are the way to go.

LOIS: *As I dressed Annie, even when she was an infant, I'd say, "Push your arm in." It was one of our first, albeit rudimentary, games. When she was less than eight weeks old, I was shocked to discover her little arms pushing at my command. But then, "Puuuush" was the first word she'd ever heard.*

The best game we found for dressing is "Where's Baby?" When you pull an article of clothing over her head, hold it for a second and say, "Where did my baby go?" As you pull it off, say *"There* she is." Act genuinely surprised. Do it every time. The baby isn't as jaded as you are and doesn't tire of this kind of babble. This game works for sleeves and socks, too.

And there's always the "Hokey Pokey" to sing as you manipulate her head into a shirt, her arms into sleeves, and her legs into pants:

You put your right arm in _(move her arm)._
You take your right arm out _(ditto)._
You put your right arm in _(ditto)._
And you shake it all about _(shake her arm gently)._
You do the Hokey Pokey _(hold her fists and wiggle them simultaneously)._
And you turn yourself around _(pick up the baby and spin around with her)._
That's what it's all about.

Other games for dressing:

➤ Count, "One, two, three, POP" as you pull off a shirt or sock.

➤ Wear her hat on your head and belt out "Born Free"; dress her quickly while she lies stunned.

➤ Save a fun little bit for last, such as a kiss for her fingers as they come through her sleeve or a clap of her feet once her socks are on.

As they near one year, babies may go through a stage during which they resist being dressed. Try "One for you, one for Teddy" as you take turns putting clothes on the baby and clothes on the bear. If you have to, make the game "One for you, one for me" (if you haven't gotten dressed yet yourself). Both of these methods may take a little longer, but they're more pleasant—for both of you—than dressing a screaming baby in a hammer hold.

Shoes and socks are their own challenge. When you need to get ten small toes into two socks and still have enough time and energy to get out of the house, opt for an amended version of "This Little Piggy":

This little piggy went to market _(wiggle her big toe)._
This little piggy stayed home _(wiggle the next one)._
This little piggy had roast beef _(wiggle the middle toe)._
This little piggy had none _(wiggle the next to last one)._
And this little piggy went wee wee wee into the sock _(wiggle the littlest toe as you bring the sock down over her foot)._

Having the child relatively immobile (already in her car seat or stroller, for example) is another game plan. Soon your child will catch on that shoes and socks mean going out—a real incentive. Jenny, once she could cruise, would find her footwear and bring it to her parents to indicate that it was time to hit the road.

Splish-Splash: Babies and Baths

Babies are rarely lukewarm about baths; they either love them or they don't. If it turns out that yours does, get ready for lots of fun. If she doesn't, you'll have to pull some rabbits out of your hat.

GENNY: *Kara loved taking a bath. Then she hated taking a bath. After a period of nightly ordeals, she tried to climb into the tub herself. Now she loves taking a bath. Sheesh.*

IN NOT-SO-DEEP WATER

For the first couple of weeks, you'll only have to give the baby a sponge bath as described in the infant care books. After her belly button heals, she's ready to graduate to a sink or baby tub. She'll probably be entranced by water and the things it can do. (If she's startled by the sound of the rushing water, just fill up the sink or tub before bringing her into the room.) Since you'll be using one of your arms to support her until she can sit up by herself, you'll have to keep games simple and, for you, one-handed. You can, however

➤ Give her something to hold on to (like a washcloth) for security.

➤ Introduce her to a washcloth mitt in the shape of an animal by singing, "The whale in the water is having fun, having fun, having fun. The whale in the water is having fun, all the livelong day."

➤ Use the spray-gun attachment on the kitchen sink (make sure to clear the cold water out of it first).

➤ Pass her hand back and forth under a trickling faucet over and over.

If all else fails, abandon the infant tub. Try bathing with her in a regular-size tub. Get in first by yourself and have a dry adult pass her to you. When the fun is over, hand her back.

Once she's an accomplished sitter, she's ready for the big tub by herself. Remember, little ones don't need head-to-toe scrubbing. A soak in the bath should be comforting and fun. Some tricks to turn the bathtime tide in your favor:

➤ Have her hold a washcloth, plastic doughnut, or bath toy for security.

➤ Gradually dip her in and out of a small amount of pleasantly warm water so she can feel it on her feet and the security of your hands at the same time.

➤ Tempt her with a new bath toy.

➤ Have her try to catch a drop of water as it falls.

➤ Bedazzle her with bubbles (use one of the mild brands made specifically for children, and check with your pediatrician first). You can keep a bubble bath bubbly if you whisk the water occasionally.

➤ Affix an unbreakable mirror at her eye level. After all, if the baby in the mirror can handle a bath, so can she.

➤ Try a tub seat, which may reduce that slip-slidey feeling. (By and large, however, we found them hard to get babies in and out of.)

➤ Put up a bathtub activity center (they attach with suction cups, which hold best when wetted first).

➤ Try bathing her with one of her pals.

➤ Give her a washcloth of her own to play with. All babies suck on them; it's okay.

Come shampoo time, if your baby allows it, simply hold her securely, tip her back, and have at it. Be swift. If your baby doesn't like being leaned back, you're going to have to get her used to water in her face. Teach her to hold her breath by using a method that many swimming instructors recommend for infants. Count to three and blow in the baby's face. The counting works as a signal and the blowing makes her reflexively hold her breath. Then, quickly and gently pour a small amount of warm water over her head and shampoo. Use the same technique to rinse.

RUBBER DUCKY AND FRIENDS: BEST BATH TOYS

If we had to elect a most versatile bath toy, the winner would be a plastic cup. It floats when it's empty, sinks when it's full. The baby can pour into it or out of it. She can fill it with other toys or, to most parents' dismay, drink out of it. She can wear one on her head (Molly looked like Jackie Kennedy with her little blue basin on her head).

When it comes to buying tub toys, you needn't look for a package designation screaming that this is an official bath toy. Anything that engages a baby's efforts to use her eyes, arms, hands, and fingers is bound to be a hit. Lots of household items and toys meant for other sorts of play qualify. If it's safe and won't get damaged by the water, it's fine. Remember this when you find yourself at Aunt Trina's without, you think, a single bath toy. Introduce them one at a time so the baby has plenty of room for herself.

Our recommendations:

➤ A rubber duck. Make sure it floats and is airtight (otherwise it will list to one side, and we can't have that). The soft vinyl ones make excellent teethers. (Sam had a duck that Molly preferred to her own because the head on Sam's was smaller than on hers and therefore fit entirely in her mouth.) The Playskool Ernie model is just ducky (sorry).

➤ Aquatic animals with moveable parts and boats with passengers are a big hit. Clear plastic balls that contain moving parts are nifty, too.

➤ Pouring toys: plastic watering cans, bottles, yogurt or margarine containers, ladles, strainers, measuring cups and spoons—all these make for long-lasting fun. Poke holes in a cup and you have a rainmaker.

➤ Sponge blocks are fun to stack, float, and topple. Put them away for a few months if your baby can't resist biting them. Ordinary sponges and Nerf balls are fun, too.

➤ Bath activity centers. These stick to, or loop over, the side of the tub and have various activities such as water wheels and spouting whales.

➤ Squirting toys. Tee hee. The baby can't work them yet, but Mommy and Daddy can. Bulb syringes and squirt and spray bottles make some babies squeal in delight. Make sure to aim low.

➤ Bath stickers. Made of vinyl or foam, they come shaped like farm animals, family members, and alphabets. Older babies will be able to stick them to the sides of the tub and peel them off again.

➤ Bubbles—the kind that come in a jar with a wand. By the end of the year, the baby may be able to blow through the wand herself.

T I P   ➤   Most plastic bath toys can be run through the dishwasher (top rack). And throw sponge toys away (or boil them) every few months, since bacteria breeds on them.

WATER MUSIC

No bath is complete without a song or three. Our top ten favorite bathtime songs are (see the "Words to Songs" appendix for some lyrics):

➤ "Rub a Dub Dub, Three Men in a Tub"

➤ "Splish-Splash"

➤ "Rubber Duckie"

➤ "This Is the Way We Wash Our . . ." (ears, toes, hands)

➤ "Row, Row, Row Your Boat"

➤ "Sailing, Sailing"

➤ "There's a Little White Duck"

➤ "Tiny Bubbles"

➤ "Raffi's Bathtime Song"

➤ "There's a Hippo in My Bathtub"

You may have a little one who thinks bathtime is the best fun in the world. Go ahead, give her two baths a day if you both enjoy it. Some kick their legs in the air and gurgle happily with every diaper change, so prolong changing time any way you can. Let the baby-care chores that your baby enjoys be fun on their own, and save the toys, tricks, and games for when she wriggles and rants and wants no part of the task at hand. Be inventive, work fast, and remember that you can always choose to try to do what you need to do—change her, dress her, bathe her—later.

2

DOMESTIC BLISS

Spending Time at Home with a Baby

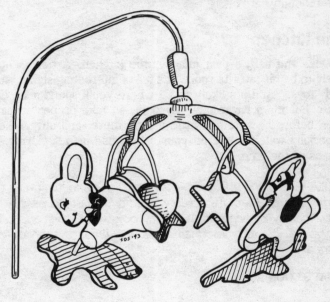

With a new baby, you're bound to spend far more time at home than ever before. You'll wake up some mornings and think, "How will I possibly get through this endless day within these four walls?" The first trick is deceptively simple: take it one chunk at a time. Break the day down into segments like: until lunchtime (yours, not the baby's), during naptime, until dinnertime, etc. While the day still may not fly by, it'll move a bit faster.

An important trick is to remember that this is your day, too. It will take some strategy and compromise to go about your business, baby in tow; most newborns, lap babies, and sitting babies will happily go along with your plans if their very basic needs are met. Crawlers and cruisers are amenable as well, as long as they have diversions and some time to stretch their legs along the way.

In this chapter, you'll find our tried-and-true solutions to spending time at home and amusing a baby. We've arranged them room by room and by developmental stage within each room. (But don't forget that your own instincts and experience in the land of amusement will kick in to guide you once the initial shock of parenthood wears off.)

The Kitchen

Once the baby's past infancy, the kitchen, Action Central, is likely to be his favorite room. It's full of interesting sights, sounds, and "toys." And it's likely to be where you'll spend a lot of your time. But it's a hazardous playroom, so take proper precautions even before he sets one little foot in there, and always keep an especially watchful eye on your baby while he's exploring, which means all the time.

PAULA: *One of the smartest things I ever did was to turn over a cabinet to my children. I kept it stocked with colorful plastic cups, bowls, and baby-friendly kitchen stuff. When my boys were sitting and crawling, they were able to amuse themselves with these toys while I cooked dinner.*

WHAT'S COOKING

Among the very first distinctions your baby will learn is the difference between hot and cold. He'll discover that it applies to what he eats and drinks, his bathwater, stoves, radiators, and, later on, the weather. Teach this valuable lesson via several games you play often; repetition is the way he'll learn. You can touch something hot for a second and make a big show of pulling your hand away while you say, "Hot" over and over. Or show him the steam that rises from anything hot, again repeating the word *hot*. Let him alternately touch something warm and something cold as you say "Hot" and "Cold" to give him a safe tactile lesson about temperature variation.

The *N* Word

The baby who constantly hears the word *no* begins to ignore it. Therefore, save it for truly important situations such as fireplaces and steep stairs. When you come upon situations in which you want to discourage the baby's behavior, try these alternatives instead of *no:*

➤ "Hot" said with a firm voice should accompany your stopping a little hand reaching for the stove or radiator.

➤ "Careful" works well to indicate he's nearing the edge of something.

➤ "Fragile" is good for delicate items and new parents' nerves (Hedy warned "Glass" when Molly approached anything breakable).

➤ "Danger" can be invoked in a grave tone when the baby's focus is an electrical cord, or such.

➤ "Yucky" discourages snacking on dust balls, lint, and the like.

➤ When your little one is dropping Cheerios into the toilet, hold his fist firmly and say, in a normal, explanatory tone, "Cheerios are food. They are for eating, not for the toilet." Then engage him with a toy or suitable game.

➤ Similarly, when he's old enough to learn not to put things in his mouth, say, "Toys are for playing, food is for eating."

Careful babyproofing is one tactic parents can use to minimize the number of nos. (Consult any infant care book for babyproofing tips and then apply your common sense.) Some of us went to great lengths to remove dangers, others did not. Make your decisions according to your sense of your child's behavior and your own preferences, keeping in mind that you want to create a welcoming environment for your baby.

LAURIE: *Anna's dad does a special blender dance before letting it loose so Anna pays attention to him and looks forward to the noise. Your baby may never come to like the noisier sounds of a kitchen, but he'll adjust if they're not sprung on him.*

To keep your baby both stimulated and to give you a moment to stir the stew, you can engage a baby's senses in numerous playful ways:

➤ Pass a bottle of vanilla extract under his nose.

➤ Let him smell a whole banana before you serve him the mashed version.

➤ Make him a set of drums out of pots, plastic bowls, and pie tins and a couple of wooden spoons. Demonstrate.

➤ Place metal measuring spoons in a cookie tin. Put Cheerios in a sealed plastic container. Give him several of these "maracas" with which to experiment.

➤ Put a whole bunch of little kitchen "toys" in a box or paper bag. He'll take each item out, inspect it, discard it, come back to it, wave it, hammer with it, rebag it, and so on.

T I P ➤ Several of us ran out and bought magnetic letters for our kids as soon as they could sit steadily on the kitchen floor. There they were on the fridge. There they were on the floor. There they went, under the fridge. As our babies couldn't really manipulate them successfully, we all put them away for a year or more.

THE MAGIC OF MEALTIME

It's an age-old argument: Should babies be allowed to play with their food? Well, they certainly don't care about nutrition. What they care about is fun and, to babies, food is fun stuff. Baby foods squish like clay, color like paint, draw like crayons. They fly nicely, too. If you can tolerate it, allow your baby to play with his first foods (maybe with a nix on the flying aspect).

Once your little gourmand has graduated from rice cereal and purees, you can start experimenting with "real" foods. (Check with your pediatrician, of course.) The easier and more fun the food is for him to handle, the better he'll like it.

LAURIE: *Anna wouldn't eat from a spoon. Unless she could pick up her food herself, she wanted no part of mealtime. In our house, even oatmeal became a finger food, which was yucky, but it worked.*

Food cut into shapes (use cookie-cutters) pleases the almost-one set. Here's a list of what worked best with our kids:

➤ macaroni and pasta (especially spaghetti, wagon-wheels, spirals, sea shells) and filled pasta (tortellini, ravioli)

➤ chicken nuggets and fish sticks (you can make your own)

➤ tofu cut in small squares or other shapes

➤ whole peas, broccoli florets (trees), steamed carrots, and avocado chunks

➤ french fries or lumpy mashed potatoes

➤ cut-up kiwi, halved grapes, a whole peeled apple, pieces of banana, berries, pineapple, chunks of melon, clementine sections, and raisins

➤ toast or French toast cut in small pieces

➤ frozen bagels (which make excellent teething rings)

➤ crackers, pretzels, breadsticks, and rice cakes (especially the miniature ones)

➤ dry cereal (a kind that a baby can pick up easily)

➤ cubed fruit-flavored gelatin

GAMES AT THE TABLE

Just as parents wonder whether they should allow their child to play with his food, they question whether they should resort to tricks to get their kids to eat. It's not a good idea to force a baby to eat when he's not hungry. But not all small children are eager to chow down the moment you plunk them in their high chairs. To get a baby in the right frame of mind, try these techniques:

➤ Show him the picture on the bottom of the bowl, mug, or plate.

➤ Give him his own spoon. It amuses him while you feed him, and he can practice feeding himself.

➤ Attach a toy with a suction cup to the tray of the high chair.

➤ Distract him with a child's placemat (some are musical).

➤ Let him dip finger foods (or his fingers) into sour cream, applesauce, or yogurt.

➤ Invite another baby over and have them face off over their plates.

➤ Change the scenery: turn his high chair a different way, try feeding him in his walker (lock the wheels), or have a picnic in a park. Remove the high-chair tray and push the chair close to the table. If your baby loves sitting in the clip-on seats many restaurants provide, consider investing in one for home use.

➤ Engage the baby in cleanup by giving him a wet washcloth. Even if he only sucks on it, he'll clean his face in the process.

The Family Room

Wherever the adults spend most of their time (in the family room, den, living room, whatever you call it) is where the baby will want to spend his time, too.

Newborns are content almost anywhere, and infants will probably be happy in a playpen, but crawlers, cruisers, and walkers gravitate to spaces designated and outfitted as their own. You can create an inviting play area by emptying a low drawer, cabinet, or shelf and filling it with an ever-changing supply of toys and books. Keep the baby's stuff clustered in that corner and he'll come to see it as his own.

Other ways you can transform the family room into babyland:

➤ Hang a mobile if your newborn will spend a lot of time here.

➤ Leave toys or propped-up books on shelves at the baby's eye level. Crawlers, cruisers, and walkers get a kick out of discovering these treasures.

➤ Set up a safe but challenging obstacle course using sofa cushions and ottomans.

➤ Put a sheet, bath towel, or blanket over a low table or over two chairs placed back-to-back to make a tent or clubhouse if your baby is not easily scared.

MEDIA AMUSEMENTS: TV FOR TOTS

Don't be afraid to turn on the television; babies have cultivated neither an attention span nor an interest in program content. The sound tracks, however, if not too loud or abrasive, may entertain them. Some babies pay close attention to the hard-driving lead music for the evening news.

"Sesame Street" and "Mr. Rogers' Neighborhood" probably won't prove hugely entertaining to your baby until, at the earliest, late in his first year. They may never be his first choices. But the music might grab the baby's attention, or he might be riveted by the vivid moving colors.

We all believe that it's a good idea, sometime in this first year, for parents to discuss their feelings about the baby's TV diet with one another and map out a general policy. It's an issue much more easily dealt with before the baby develops a fondness for any particular program than after.

This is also a good time to get in the habit of screening television programs and videos geared for toddlers before letting your child watch. The most musical ones might interest a baby in the last months of his first year (see Chapter 6, "For a Song," for further discussion of this topic). If you have a video camera, watching tapes of family get-togethers starring You Know Who will entertain him, too.

Step by Step

Stairs and steps intrigue babies. Once he starts to crawl, you'll have trouble keeping him away from them. Now that he's got locomotion down, his next challenge is to climb and gain height. In fact, once he's mastered the skill, he may want to do little else but crawl upstairs. He may, however, be somewhat perplexed about how to get down again.

There are a couple of games you can use to help teach a baby— even a sitting baby—about step safety. Position him on the top step on his tummy, his hands on the top step, his feet pointing down. Guide his feet to the next step and help him slide his tummy and hands down. Say a funny word (boink, for instance) in a funny voice as he lands safely. Or recite one line of a nursery rhyme, with each step. With older babies, you can count each step.

When he reaches the bottom, be sure to lavish sincere praise. Give the game a name like Feet First or Tushy First so you can use it again when he's learning to get off a sofa or bed. Make sure to pick a name that you won't mind yelling to him across a playground as he's preparing to slither down headfirst from some piece of equipment you hadn't thought he'd be able to find his way onto in the first place.

Another method is to come down stairs sitting down. Sit the baby on the top step and have him hold on to it. Point his feet toward the next step down. Push his bottom forward till he plunks down onto the next step; his hands should come along automatically. Molly's grandma taught her to yell "Bump!" with each step.

Try both ways with your baby and see which he likes better. No matter how great a time you both had learning this game, don't expect your baby to remember it the next time. Stay close by when your mountain climber takes to the steps. If you haven't already installed a safety gate, now's the time. Make sure to replace it as soon as you are finished with the game.

The Nursery

In spite of the fabulous layouts you've seen in magazines and at baby furniture shops, babies don't really need much in the way of space or equipment for entertainment. The most important thing is to make a pleasant, comfortable spot for your baby that's a safe and serviceable play area.

One way to build play into the baby's quarters is to hang a wallpaper border or to paint a stencil at crib height. (Check the remnant bin at the wallpaper store; a leftover end might be just enough for one wall.) While you're in the baby's room, you can invent stories about the characters or use them in the old standbys. Who says those particular bears aren't *the* three bears?

Or use stickers, book jackets, wrapping paper, pictures from magazines, or photographs to customize your own storyland. Libraries and children's bookstores sometimes have surplus posters they'll happily give away. The little one will come to know and love his first cast of characters. One morning you'll wake up to hear the baby gurgling away, deep in conversation with his favorite critter.

If you have the room and the funds, buy a comfortable rocking chair. At first you'll use it for feedings, catnaps, and soothing. Later it'll be the perfect venue for lap games. Eventually it'll become home base for story time.

Hang mobiles. The musical ones, especially, really entertain some babies, which can make falling asleep and waking up a more pleasant time for you both. In a few months, your baby will start looking forward to the music when he sees your hand move toward the winding mechanism. He'll enjoy hearing you hum the tune even when you're elsewhere.

Points to consider as you're buying a mobile and deciding where to hang it:

➤ When placing mobiles, remember that infants naturally hold their heads to the side, so hang mobiles to one side, not directly over the baby.

➤ Look for mobiles with the dangling objects (clowns, bears, whatever) facing down so your baby can look them in the eye.

➤ Check the winding mechanism on musical mobiles; you want a reasonably quiet one so it won't rouse a sleepy baby.

➤ Make sure the tune is one you won't mind listening to ninety-five times a day.

➤ Just because your baby can grab the mobile once he can pull himself up, don't remove it entirely. Just hang it on a wall or ceiling so it's out of harm's way. Or cut the toys off the mobile and give them to the baby as, well, toys.

Our favorites are the high-contrast Wimmer Ferguson black-and-white mobile (about $15) and Dakin's primary-colored Bears Over the Rainbow model (about $50).

Put an unbreakable mirror in the baby's crib. Once they can push up on their forearms at two to three months, babies adore looking at the most captivating face of all—their own.

SIMPLE MIRROR GAMES

Don't think just in terms of the baby's crib mirror. There are all sorts of games to play in front of mirrors anywhere:

➤ Hold the baby so he's facing the mirror and say, "Look, there's George" (point to his reflection in the mirror) and "Look, there's Mommy" (point to your reflection).

➤ Make silly faces at the baby in the mirror.

➤ Make funny sounds like raspberries, whistles, and clucks while you both watch in the mirror. Or watch yourselves laugh.

➤ Put one hat on you and another on the baby. Switch them. Switch them back. Cover your face with one. Cover his face briefly with one.

➤ Name the baby's facial features as you touch them on the real baby, then name them as you touch them on the mirror baby.

LAURIE: *Anna was endlessly fascinated with her reflection from the get-go. She found it hysterically amusing to try out new expressions and sounds in front of the mirror.*

———————

T I P ➤ As wonderful a distraction as a mirror can be, avoid showing the baby what he looks like in full cry. You don't want him to distance himself from his own emotions.

The Bedroom

Rolling around and getting comfy on a big squishy bed is a great game for babies of all ages. And it's a delightful activity that the entire family can enjoy.

GENNY: *The first game to get a laugh out of Kara every time was one we started playing on the bed when she was just shy of two months. I'd straddle her on my hands and knees and bounce, bounce, bounce. She'd gurgle. What ecstasy.*

There are lots of ways to play with a baby in bed:

➤ If he seems to like being diaperless, let him lie naked (on a rubber-backed sheet) to stretch, kick, and swat.

➤ Lay him on his back and gently bounce the mattress a tiny bit.

➤ Cuddle, snuggle, or massage him.

➤ Put the little one in the center of the bed and call to him from one side. Switch to the other side after he's turned his head and found you.

➤ Duck down below the mattress level and call to him. Lift your head up and say, "Boo!"

➤ Play peekaboo with the blanket or pillow.

➤ Practice new skills like rolling over and sitting up. Now watch the baby try.

➤ Practice the Feet First or Tushy First game.

➤ Make a bunker with pillows or a clubhouse with blankets.

➤ Put dolls and toys "to bed." Bounce a stuffed animal as if it were on a trampoline.

LIBBY: _We had a family ritual of "schnoogling" in bed on the weekends. Whichever parent got Sam out of his crib signaled the start of the game by humming the theme from_ The Pink Panther _as he or she skulked toward the big bed and then leapt in. Sam has always enjoyed the silliness and the family cuddle and now initiates the game himself._

T I P ➤ If you are trying to perform some simple task that requires two hands and the baby is fussing, put him on the bed and jiggle the mattress with your foot or sit down and bounce.

Other bedroom fun, particularly useful if you're caught on a phone call or if you need to lie down for a few minutes, can be found in

➤ your empty jewelry case or bureau organizer (especially if it has interesting lids and drawers)

➤ bangle bracelets

➤ hair ornaments or smooth plastic hair curlers

➤ hats

- ➤ makeup brushes and hair combs

- ➤ purses, pocketbooks, briefcases, tote bags, and a bunch of stuff to put in them

- ➤ an empty hamper or laundry basket

- ➤ the entire sock drawer

- ➤ an unbreakable mirror

- ➤ bureau handles that rattle

LAURIE: *I could always buy a few minutes in the bedroom by giving Anna the run of a drawer containing a collection of purses and a few hats. She'd drape purses over her shoulders and perch floppy hats on her head. Try sitting a prewalker in front of a full-length mirror with a bunch of accessories and see what happens.*

PAULA: *My makeup and perfume shelf has always been a focus of my boys' curiosity. I collected and washed empty cosmetic and perfume containers and made an exact replica of my own makeup kit for George. We'd share the mirror and do our faces together in the morning.*

The Home Office

No matter what safety precautions you take, some rooms are not great play areas for babies. Home offices fall into this category. There are loads of dangerous, expensive, mess-making baby tempters. Those of us who had our own desks or offices at home found it best to make them off-limits from the beginning.

Still, sometimes business cannot wait. So:

➤ Keep a basket of small toys near the phone for just such emergencies.

➤ If you have a swivel chair, rock back and forth with the baby in your lap.

➤ Let him tap on the keys of your (turned off) typewriter or computer keyboard.

➤ Use the Telephone Fake-Out game (described in Chapter 1, "Basic Training").

➤ Hand him some unimportant file cards as if you were entrusting him with Swiss bank notes. "Oooh. What's this vitally important document?"

➤ Give him a magazine, catalog, or junk mail to "read."

➤ Give him a cup of unsharpened pencils and let him dump them out and fill the cup again. (Be forewarned: the erasers he puts in his mouth will never erase again.)

➤ Make a finger puppet by using a ballpoint pen to draw a face on your finger or a pencil eraser cap. Put on a silent puppet show.

➤ Let him push the buttons of your calculator or adding machine.

➤ Keep some perforated ends of computer paper around so you can shower him with a ticker tape parade.

➤ Keep some crayons in your pencil cup so he can work alongside you if his fine motor coordination is sufficiently advanced.

➤ Rip off the front panel of an envelope with a window so he can look through it at you and you at him.

Apartment Life

Raising a baby in an apartment has its ups and downs (literally). Even though you're probably working with less space than you would have in a house, the big advantage is the plenitude of neighbors very close by. The odds of finding playmates (for you *and* the baby) are in your favor. Make friends with other parents in the building even if you wouldn't otherwise seek them out. You *do* have babies in common, and this makes for a strong bond.

It's fun when you and your baby have playmates you'll see, if only in passing on the elevator, just about every day. On nasty or cold days, you won't have to wrestle on shoes and a snowsuit to have a play date. (You might not even need to get out of your bathrobe.) On days when you find yourselves with time to spare, you can often link up with neighbors on the spur of the moment.

Lobbies, elevators, stairs, doormen, and laundry rooms are the other pluses of apartment buildings. If yours has a playroom, courtyard, or recreation center, consider yourself especially fortunate. (Once you're a member of your building's baby circuit, you can gauge others' interest in putting together a playroom or chipping in on a large piece of equipment.) When you can't look at your four walls another minute, go on a building tour:

➤ Even little ones enjoy the sensation of moving up and down on an elevator. Older babies are intrigued by the buttons and illuminated panels of numbers.

➤ Once your baby's ready for stairs, let him loose on the interior building stairs (with you right behind).

➤ Pay a visit to the doorman or elevator operator just for fun.

➤ Let the baby try out his push and pull toys in the hallway or lobby (depending on the level of soundproofing and the tolerance of your neighbors).

➤ Go down to the laundry room and watch the clothes go around in the dryer.

➤ Go up to the roof (assuming it's safe) and get a bird's-eye view of your neighborhood.

➤ Visit an older resident, especially one who doesn't get out much.

LIBBY: *Sam learned up and down, open and close, numbers and the letter B (for basement) from the elevator panel in our building. He started shaking hands and giving high and low fives with our doormen. And best of all, he learned about homemade cookies from Mrs. Rosenthal in Apartment 44.*

Animal Magnetism

A pet can be a wonderful playmate for your baby. And a baby can be a wonderful playmate for your pet. The trick is to acquaint them with each other in ways that take their limitations into account. Proper training is crucial, so ask your vet and consult pet-care and baby-care books for the ground rules.

It may turn out that your pet shows little interest in the baby. Laurie's cats couldn't have cared less about Anna's debut. Blazer, Lois's dog, however, moped around the house for days, believing that the sudden changes in the household meant that she'd done something wrong. Every pet-owning parent we consulted stressed that you must give the pet as much attention as you can to avoid jealousy.

Avoid pet toys and baby toys that look alike, or you will all have trouble keeping track of which is whose. You don't want the baby to teethe on the dog's rubber rattle, and you don't want the cat to snatch the baby's toy mouse.

HEDY: _The first couple of times we chastized our retriever, Sam, in front of Libby's son, the boy would start to cry. We quickly caught on that the boy thought we were talking to him, not the dog. Now we call the four-legged one Sam the Dog and the two-legged one Sam the Boy._

Assuming that the pet shows an interest in your baby, meaning he doesn't remove himself every time the baby draws near, you'll need to start teaching the baby how to handle the pet. (This is also a good way to start teaching a baby how to handle other children.) To make a game out of helping the baby learn the magic word "gently," take the baby's hand in yours and stroke the pet together so he can feel what "gently" means as he hears the word. You can practice on stuffed animals, your own body, and the baby's body. "Put love in your hand" is how Lois explained it to Annie, who now charmingly repeats the message to her playmates.

One game that a trainer recommended to Lois to help foster amicable relations between Blazer and Annie was to have Annie leave a treat in Blazer's bowl while the dog looked on. Blazer associated Annie's little fingers with giving rather than taking away. (Do this only when the pet's food dish is empty, when you are there, and with your own animal.)

LOIS: _When you and your child visit someone with a dog, always ask your hosts to remove the dog's bowl until you leave. Even the most gentle dog may become aggressive if a baby meddles with its food._

Keeping fish certainly has less potential for mishap than other pets. For the same reasons they are entranced by windows, babies love to gaze at fish tanks. Colorful aquarium toys, streams of bubbles, and shiny moving fish may command your baby's attention long before he's ready for television.

PAULA: *Our aquarium has given George great pleasure. He has loved watching the fish since he could sit up. He became an enthusiastic fish feeder when he neared one. We had to change the tank water only twice as a result of overfeeding. Among his first words were "fffeeeeed fffish."*

I'm Exhausted, How About You: Quiet Games for You Both

A baby's day (for most babies, anyway) has a definite rhythm. It may take you awhile to figure out what that rhythm is, but it is, no doubt, there. (Just when you figure it out, however, it will change. Typical. Cruel, but typical.) Some children have uncannily accurate body clocks and will settle down at the same time every day. Some act like whirling dervishes until they collapse in an exhausted, fretful heap.

SETTLING DOWN, SETTLING IN

It's best to head babies off before they get to the overtired point of no return. When you sense the time has come, announce to the baby that it's quiet time and help the child wind down. Some people like to initiate quiet time by putting toys away. It should be a special time, a time the baby looks forward to, so don't wait until you're tired or angry to announce it. Quiet time is a time for intimacy, cuddling, and relaxing, low-key games such as:

➤ Telling stories, reading books, and singing lullabies or other quiet songs.

➤ Focusing on a quiet lap game (see Chapter 4, "Fun and Games," for a list).

➤ Rocking in a rocking chair or swing.

➤ Taking a warm bath.

➤ Giving the baby a massage.

➤ Lying down together. If you like, talk quietly to the baby (a kind of verbal lullaby) about the things you did so far that day or the things you'll do later. He won't understand the words, but your soothing tones might help him drop off.

T I P   ➤ When it's quiet time, check to see if the things you might want (the phone, the remote control, tissues, a blanket, brownies, reading material) are close at hand; if the baby falls asleep on you, you may not want to move.

CREATING ISLANDS OF PEACE FOR YOURSELF

The changes a baby brings to your life and to your home weigh heavily on a new parent—especially on the parent who spends the most time with the baby. As far as getting through each day goes and having some fun while you do it, it's important to take some time to yourself. This will seem next to impossible during the first weeks when it's hard to focus on anything but the baby. But try anyway. As the baby gets older, you'll invent your own strategies to give yourself the breathing space you'll need.

When the baby is napping, take the time to restore yourself. Turn off "The Teddybears' Picnic" and do something that makes *you* happy. Read a magazine. Linger over a cup of tea. Write a letter. Tinker with a personal project. Put a corny old movie into the VCR. Take a bath. Here's a novel idea: NAP.

You can also spend a free moment or two considering that the baby isn't the only one accomplishing new feats. Think of the new skills *you've* mastered in the last few months:

➤ You can do a remarkable number of chores that require fine motor skills—in the dark, in nanoseconds, simultaneously.

➤ You can take a catnap standing up on a bus, wearing the baby in his carrier, while holding a bag of groceries, and wake feeling oddly refreshed.

➤ You can extend an open hand toward any baby's mouth when his cheeks look suspiciously full and accept whatever comes out without gagging.

➤ You can find the infant department in seconds—whenever you're shopping for anything anywhere.

➤ You've discovered that pureed apricots taste mighty fine over chocolate fudge ice cream after 4 A.M. feedings.

➤ You've learned every Raffi lyric and all the characters' names on "Sesame Street." (And your Cookie Monster imitation brings down the house during play group.)

➤ You've accepted food smears on your clothes as a fashion statement.

➤ You and your relatives, neighbors, friends, and pediatrician have established fifty adjectives to describe poop (and, yes, we know, Dr. Freud, "dirty" is not one of them).

➤ You can take a shower in seventeen seconds with the curtain open while distracting your baby with your lathered-up conehead, singing "Wild Thing," and dancing the Pony all at once.

➤ You can eat out because you've learned to control dawdling waiters with withering looks that say, "This innocent blossom might look like a baby but it's really a time bomb with a very short fuse so *feed me . . . now.*"

Now, give yourself a pat on the back for being such a caring, loving parent.

3

OUT AND ABOUT

Finding Your Way from Here to There

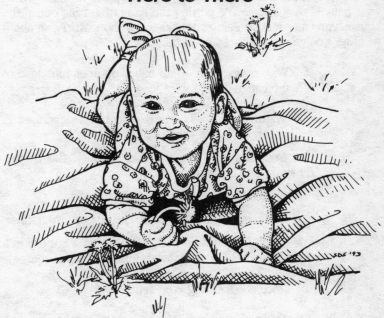

Going outside and taking a look around is a wonderful, simple, and affordable game. If you think it's the same old, same old, you've never been around the block with a baby. Think of it as your baby might: The world is brand new and every inch of it is absolutely fascinating to your munchkin; watching her take it all in makes every step of the route you've trodden a zillion times seem like a trip into uncharted territory. Let your baby be your tour guide.

Don't reject the idea of going somewhere because your little one *might* raise a fuss and disturb others. She might not. She might be a perfect angel from start to finish. And if she does fall victim to a crank attack, you can usually remove yourselves from the situation until the storm subsides. Be brave, and remember that yours isn't the first baby to cry in public.

Garden of Delights

Your backyard, porch, or deck is the best place to start. While your baby is new and you're getting the hang of getting out of the house, you can practice going somewhere without worrying about whether you've remembered everything.

 With a newborn or lap baby, outdoor fun close to home can include:

➤ Nature tours, like the house tours described in Chapter 1, "Basic Training."

➤ Watching the sun shimmer through the leaves, listening to birds (or traffic).

➤ Swinging in a hammock or porch swing.

➤ Watching for birds in a bird feeder or bird bath.

➤ Taking an outdoor bath together on a hot day in a kiddie pool (with a big towel close at hand, of course).

 Once she's sitting, you can:

➤ Bring some toys with you into the wading pool.

➤ Position the baby at the bottom of a ramp (a large piece of cardboard placed over a stoop works fine) and roll cars or balls down to her.

➤ Attach a safety belt to a wagon or wheelbarrow, put in some pillows or blankets, and take her for a gentle ride.

➤ Take her out while it's raining or snowing so she can feel raindrops or snowflakes on her face.

➤ Blow bubbles toward her (hold the wand yourself so her fingers don't get soapy; bring a wet washcloth just in case).

To appeal to a crawler:

➤ Take her out while it's raining or snowing and let her try to catch the raindrops or snowflakes.

➤ Blow bubbles away from her and let her catch them.

➤ "Garden" with her shovel and watering can; plant bulbs or seeds.

➤ Show her a pine cone or dandelion and go hunting for others.

➤ Play in the soil with toy bulldozers and dump trucks.

Outdoor activities for cruisers capitalize on their mobility:

➤ Show her a little gate or door for her to open, close, and go through to her heart's content. Obviously, make sure the mechanism isn't so springy that it'll pinch her fingers.

➤ Give her a frozen fruit juice pop or some other fun, messy treat and watch her get sloppy. Show her her colored tongue in a mirror.

➤ Put a toy in her stroller and suggest she take it for a ride.

➤ Use fat chalk to color the pavement or "paint" with a pot of water and a brush.

➤ Give her a cupful of bird seed to pour into a feeder and then watch for birds or squirrels.

➤ Bring her push toy or ride-on toy out for a spin.

➤ Save stale bread or broken crackers and feed the squirrels, fish, ducks, or birds.

Invisible Toys

There you are out in the world having a wonderful time with your baby. But then . . . you get stuck in traffic. There's a long line to get into the museum you've just traveled forty-five minutes to visit. Your arsenal of toys, songs, and games is depleted. You're both edgy.

That's when you bring out the invisible toys, the playthings that aren't truly "toys" but that can be counted on for fun nevertheless. Your body counts as a toy (see Chapter 4, "Fun and Games," and the "Words to Songs" appendix for games to play with fingers, hands, toes, and so on). And you can anthropomorphize anything— a sock, glove, eyeglasses—for an impromptu puppet show.

Personal belongings to use in a pinch are:

➤ your scarf, perfect for peekaboo

➤ your clothes (nubby winter coats, bumpy corduroy, etc.)

➤ your wallet, which the baby will love to empty, pausing only to inspect the photographs

➤ your watch (if it's shock resistant or one of those rubberized, waterproof models); if it makes beeping noises on demand, so much the better

➤ a pocket calculator

➤ a pager (especially if it can be made to beep)

➤ bangle bracelets, oversized earrings

➤ your keys

➤ a purse mirror

➤ barrettes, ponytail holders, etc.

➤ fragrant hand cream, perfume, or makeup (good for sniffing)

In the car, try:

➤ a flashlight

➤ the ice scraper (draw a face on it with a marker)

➤ the remote control for the garage door

➤ a map that you don't mind seeing destroyed

Infant swings, sandboxes, slides, playhouses, and gyms are great backyard fun (they're fun indoors, too, if you have the room). Before investing, test drive these amusements at a local playground or toy store to see if your baby is ready for them.

Outings

You might as well face it. Getting out of the house is going to take longer when you're getting two people ready instead of one. But keeping to certain habits (and having reasonable expectations) will help make your expeditions fun:

➤ Keep the baby's diaper bag packed with the essentials so you can just add items you'll need for that particular trip.

➤ Keep a couple of dollars buried in the bag so that when you leave the house without your wallet you still have some cash. Same with an extra house key.

➤ Only bring along as much as you're comfortable toting.

➤ Keep a couple of toys or books hidden in the diaper bag to use as distractions. Change them occasionally.

➤ Always pack a bright bandanna. It folds smaller than, dries faster than, and can be tied to your stroller more easily than a cloth diaper. You can use it as an impromptu bib, sunshade, washcloth, or peekaboo aid.

➤ Allow yourself lots of time.

➤ Remember that most trips are not essential; it's not the end of the world if you don't get to where you were going. Try again later or on another day.

CHOOSING THE RIGHT TRANSPORT

Infant carriers, slings, and backpacks are ideal for getting around with babies. Having a baby close to your head makes it easy to talk and point things out to her. If you are going far, staying out for a while, or find the baby too heavy to carry, go with the stroller. At first, while her field of vision is fairly shallow, use plastic links to hang a favorite rattle over the seat.

Once she's passed the six- to eight-month mark, you can encourage her to look beyond the stroller bar by pointing things out as you go by. (Don't take the toys away, though; she'll probably still like playing with them.) By the end of the year, she'll be pointing out dogs, fire trucks, and other fascinating sights to you.

You shouldn't think of your adventure together strictly as getting from point A to point B. Take advantage of serendipitous opportunities. When you pass by a mossy rock, stop to touch and smell it. When you pass by a fabric store, clean her hands and let her feel the different textures. When you hear an unusual sound (an airplane, waterfall, or cricket), stop to listen. When you pass by a bakery, stand still long enough to get a good sniff—or go in and buy yourself a treat. Keep sensory games like these in mind as diversions when the baby is confined in a stroller or car seat and while traveling.

Playground Pleasantries

You may not think there's anything much for a less-than-one-year-old baby to do at a playground. Wrong. There are plenty of opportunities for her to observe other children, practice her new skills, and explore. But the biggest attraction of a playground is a fresh supply of playmates—for both of you.

 Newborns can do anything at the playground that they can do at home—watch you, look around, snooze, watch you some more. The fun in a trip to the playground at this age is the change of scenery, the fresh air, and the new sensory experiences (the bells on the ice cream truck, for example).

T I P ➤ When in doubt about safety, courtesy, or playground politics, take the path of least resistance and move your baby. Don't chastize an offending child yourself if the accompanying adult is nearby and attentive. If the grown-up's not in sight and the offense is significant, such as hitting or biting, go find the adult. Try not to let the outrage over sand in your baby's eyes get the best of you.

As your baby matures, there'll be more and more for her to do. Once she can sit up, she'll actually be able to play at the playground. You can start off with:

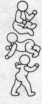

➤ Bucket swings: place the baby all the way forward in the seat (maybe with a rolled-up blanket or pillow at her back to fill the gap; you can also put two babies back-to-back in some models). Push her once very gently (from the front so she can see you). Let her swing a few times before you push again. Sing, "She flies through the air with the greatest of ease." Swing a little harder if she likes it. Tap her feet and knees with an "I got your feet, sweet, I got your knees, sneeze" rhyme. Later in the year, if she likes to go high, you can duck when she comes toward you and straighten up calling, "Peekaboo" when she swings away.

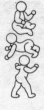

➤ The sandbox: sit in the sandbox together and watch as your brilliant baby knows exactly what to do—pick up a fistful of sand and eat it—without being taught. Take the baby's hand away from her mouth as she tries to eat the sand and say, "Sand isn't food," gently but firmly. Repeat a zillion times. Fill up a small pail or other container (yogurt cups are ideal) and see if she'll turn it over. Turn it over for her if she doesn't. Bury her hands and feet (barefoot is fine in warm weather) and play peekaboo. Pour sand over the baby's open hand or toes. Build tiny castles and let her play Ms. Destructo. (Some kids just plain don't like the feel of sand; try it again another time.)

➤ The slide: many playgrounds have small slides (no more than about four feet high) for little tykes and larger ones for bigger kids. Start on the small one. You can sit the baby on your lap and go down together. Or put the baby at the top, hold her securely around the tummy, and slide her down with a big "Whee." Or put her on her tummy and slide her down feet first. Teach her the ritual of banging her feet on the slide before coming down (the noise is deafening but babies think it's a laugh riot). Depending on the child, by eight months to a year she may be ready to go solo, provided there's a familiar face waiting at the bottom to catch her. On those rare days when a playground isn't crowded, sit the baby on the ground at the bottom of the slide and roll a ball down to her.

LIBBY: *I remember bringing Sam home from the playground when he had just learned how to sit up solo. We'd had a ball. For the first time in his life, my baby was grubby. He was a regular kid. I was ecstatic.*

 ➤ A seesaw: some playgrounds have two-seat boat- or airplane-shaped seesaws that rock gently back and forth. Once she's a daredevil cruising baby, she might like the big seesaw if you hold her securely on one end while her best pal (held by another grownup) or a sibling rides on the other. Or get on the seesaw yourself, with another grownup on the other end, and hold the babies on your lap Sing:

> See Saw Margery Daw
> Jackie has got a new master.
> He shall have but a penny a day
> Because he can't work any faster.

 ➤ Wading pool or sprinkler: if the baby likes the bathtub, she'll probably adore outdoor aquatics. If you don't mind getting wet, hold the baby in your arms and run through the sprinkler.

 ➤ Suspension bridge (a.k.a. bouncing or jumping bridge): this piece of equipment is meant for babies who can stand by themselves, but on an uncrowded day, you can try it out with a younger baby. Hold the baby in your arms and bounce on your toes. Graduate to a full-fledged jump if she seems to like it. You can sit a baby on the bridge between your feet and bounce gently, too. A crawler might like to traverse the length on her knees, a cruiser while holding onto the railing. If an older jumping bean joins your little crawler or cruiser, take yours off before she goes sky-high.

➤ Monkey bars: little ones are more interested in teething on, crawling under, and cruising around monkey bars and jungle gyms than climbing them. Steer small babies clear of older climbers who think of baby heads as handy footholds.

What Toys to Bring

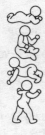

➤ bubbles

➤ sand toys—"real" ones, or just the serving spoon from a set of flatware and a couple of small plastic bowls. Other choices include sifters, funnels, strainers, molds. A general rule is the smaller the baby's hands, the smaller the container.

➤ an inflatable ball

➤ crusts of bread for squirrels and birds

➤ a squeeze bottle filled with water for flushing sandy eyes

➤ powder (which, when sprinkled on sandy fingers, toes, or bottoms, magically absorbs moisture and causes the sand to fall off)

New Frontiers: Other Places to Go with a Baby

There are plenty of other places you can go with a baby. And, no, your baby doesn't have to be "ready" for the real purpose of the destination. You and your baby, no matter how small, will find something interesting to see or do. Here are our suggestions, all of which you should keep in mind as fun expeditions while traveling, too. You'll discover your own favorites in your neck of the woods.

➤ bakeries, florists, nurseries, and lumber yards (they smell good)

➤ botanical gardens, arboretums, and sculpture gardens

➤ art museums, many of which have sculpture gardens, fountains, and other attractions that babies like; natural history museums; and children's museums

➤ churches or other buildings with stained-glass windows

➤ farmers' markets

➤ pet stores

➤ firehouses, especially those with friendly dogs

➤ police stations (there are all sorts of police vehicles, each with a siren and blinking lights)

➤ zoos

➤ aquariums (even tiny babies are entranced by fish tanks, and older ones will love seeing the sea lions fed)

➤ riding stables

➤ carousels

➤ municipal buildings with shallow flights of stairs

➤ toy stores that allow babies to play with the toys

➤ malls, especially when it's too hot, cold, or rainy to be outside but you can't stand another minute inside; the other children, waterfalls, music, displays, escalators, elevators, steps, toy stores, and carousels—all will delight babies of all ages

➤ department stores

T I P ➤ If you're on maternity or paternity leave (rather than a physical disability leave), you may want to plan a visit to your workplace. You'll get a chance to catch up with coworkers, and they'll love to ooh and aah over your baby.

Before setting out for any of these places, especially if you're going with someone else, try and do some groundwork. Find out if:

➤ it's open

➤ babies are allowed

➤ parking or public transportation is convenient

➤ strollers are permitted and if there's a best entrance for going in with one

➤ there's a central place where you can wait or return to periodically in case someone you're meeting is late

➤ there's a snack bar, water fountain, or other food service

➤ there's somewhere to sit down

➤ there are changing facilities and toilets

T I P ➤ It's always awkward when your baby buries herself in your neck just as an admirer tries to befriend her. It's even worse when she shies away from your favorite relative or closest friend. But it's also entirely normal. Don't make a big deal of it and let the baby find her own moment to surface and make eye contact.

Seasonal Outings

Try to take advantage of special events and attractions timed to coincide with changing seasons and holidays:

➤ flower shows

➤ carnivals

➤ parades

➤ marinas, which are full of unusual sights, smells, and sounds

➤ ferry rides

➤ the beach

➤ sailboat rides

➤ fairs and festivals

➤ pumpkin farms (superb photo opportunities)

➤ the skating rink (to look at the colorful skaters and listen to the music)

➤ department store holiday displays

T I P   ➤   If the weather is above freezing, below scorching, and not raining cats and dogs and your baby is in good health and dressed appropriately (dress her as her grandmother would, then take off a layer, recommends one of our pediatricians), go out.

If your baby happens to be beyond the six-month mark when her first snowfall falls, pull on your snow suits and head on out for winter games:

➤ Pull her around on a sled or a plastic tray.

➤ Use kitchen molds, cookie cutters, or sand toys to make impressions in the snow.

➤ Make mitten prints or body prints (angels) in the snow and compare them.

➤ Build "castles" in the snow and decorate them with sticks, stones, leaves, etc.

➤ Compare your footprints and look for animal tracks.

Eating Out

Your first reaction might well be, "What, are you nuts!" But eating out can actually be pleasurable for all of you. Really. Truly.

Our first tip about dining out is to feed the baby beforehand. Second is to choose a restaurant that caters to families. Most casual places that don't fit the baby-friendly description below are still fine choices. Fancy, expensive restaurants won't do. Third, avoid rush hour by dining a little on the early or late side if you can, but don't go at all during your baby's most volatile times of day.

Look for a place that

➤ uses paper tablecloths and puts crayons on the table

➤ offers balloons

➤ has a children's menu

➤ supplies high chairs, booster seats, or clip-on seats, or doesn't mind if you bring your own

➤ has kids of all ages running around and waitresses and waiters who smile at them

Even if you're going to the baby-friendliest place in the world, bring some toys: a ring of plastic keys, a busy box, a couple of favorite books, anything that's not too noisy and doesn't have lots of pieces you'll have to keep diving under the table to retrieve. Bring them out one at a time when you see her tiring of flirting with the people at the next table.

When dining with a newborn or lap baby, be prepared to eat fast and:

➤ Get a table under a working ceiling fan or by a window, both of which give her something to gaze at.

➤ Sit by a mirrored wall and play games.

➤ While you're waiting for your food, give the baby a tour: check out the bathroom and play some mirror games, belly up to the bar (if the baby doesn't mind noise) for a sip of juice or a slice of orange, and watch the blinking lights of the pinball machine or jukebox. Is there a fish tank to watch?

➤ When *your* food arrives, continue to amuse the baby by making faces, exaggerate your chewing, chat with her, and leave a big tip.

Once the baby can sit up (and is eating solids):

➤ If the baby likes what's in the bread basket, let her have it. She can snack, crush crackers, or watch you build a log cabin out of breadsticks.

➤ Do a finger dance using an overturned ashtray as a stage or get a tiny paper parasol from the bar for a Gene Kelly number.

➤ Blow through a straw at her, aiming for each of her fingers or starting at her head and working your way down her body.

➤ Go with another adult and baby and position the babies' high chairs so they can watch each other.

When she's got the greater dexterity of a cruiser:

➤ Ask for a small cup of ice cubes for her to play with. Show her how to use her spoon to stir them around.

➤ Use a napkin as a puppet or a peekaboo curtain.

➤ If there's an outdoor section, sit there. Usually

there's enough room for a crawling or cruising baby to roam and plants and shrubbery to look at (and crying doesn't seem so loud outdoors).

➤ Ball up a wet paper napkin and play tabletop soccer.

➤ Make use of paper placemats: draw pictures, make a hat, see if you remember how to do origami.

T I P   ➤ Ask that the baby's food (and the plate it is served on) not be brought piping hot. If she's hungry and her meal comes to the table too hot to eat, she' guaranteed to fuss while she waits.

I Get Around

Babies who love motion also love rides to anywhere and nowhere. To get where you need to go or for no reason at all, hop in the car, on a bus, train, subway, ferry, monorail, or whatever else passes by your house. (Some pediatricians recommend that babies not risk such exposure before they've been given the DPT vaccine at two months.) The ride itself and the sights to be found on board and en route are usually so interesting that toys from home are superfluous. However, you can make things easier for yourself if you

➤ Sing a song like "Wheels on the Bus"; tailor it to whatever mode of transportation you're on. ("The lights on the street turn red and green," "The bus on the highway goes zoom, zoom, zoom," "The driver in the Ford is a pig, pig, pig," "The engine on the train goes choo, choo, choo," etc.).

➤ Make a game out of looking out the window and talking about what you see (make sure to talk about things that are far enough ahead that the baby will be able to spot them before they're gone).

➤ If you have another adult with you, concoct a long shaggy dog story by alternating lines and using words the baby will recognize.

➤ Make up a song with gaps the baby can fill with whatever sounds or words she is able to make.

➤ Remember to use your invisible toys.

A happy baby will make you fantasize about driving cross-country from Maine to Alaska. A screaming baby can make you want to run off the road. Here are some tips for keeping an eye on the road and a hand on the wheel:

➤ Use plastic links to attach a few dangling toys (rattles, unbreakable Christmas ornaments, little busy boxes, things that will move along with the car's motion) to the car seat. The baby will learn to retrieve her toys by reeling in the links.

➤ Sing along to the radio or tape player or a cappella. Go for songs that give the baby something to do, such as "If You're Happy and You Know It" (see the "Words to Songs" appendix) and choose activities that she can do while in her car seat. Or try songs that can go on and on, like "Old MacDonald" and "There Was an Old Lady." Sing "Happy Birthday" to everyone your baby knows, grouped by family, occupation, or association.

➤ Use hand puppets, if you've got someone else in the car to work them. If you don't, make a cast of puppets by drawing little faces on your fingertips.

➤ Borrow a ten-year-old to ride in back with the baby. Next to you, kids are the best entertainment a baby could hope for.

➤ Attach a stroller toy or mini steering wheel to the car seat so she can play her favorite game: imitating you.

➤ Keep a couple of small books or toys that the baby can play with in the glove compartment. Some new parents worry about babies getting motion sickness from "reading" in a car. Not to worry. Babies don't get carsick the way older kids and adults can.

If you opt for public transportation:

➤ Count down the number of stops you have left. (When Jenny was fussing, Jil did this loudly enough so that other passengers could hear and know when to expect their reprieve.)

➤ Show the baby the route map, indicating, "This is where we live," "This is where we're going," etc. No, she won't understand, but she'll probably like the colored lines and shapes.

Where your outings take you will depend entirely on where you live. And what your baby learns from them will vary accordingly, too. Naturally, urban and rural babies will develop slightly different repertoires. City tykes will know a hook and ladder from an ambulance before they can talk. Country kids will be able to tell a John Deere from a Jane doe at sixty paces.

The point isn't where you go. Just go; you'll both have fun.

PART

II

Let the Games Begin

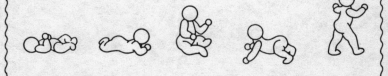

4

FUN AND GAMES

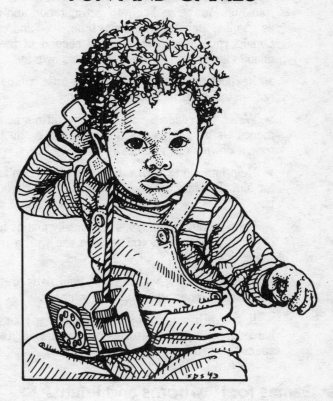

For babies, playtime is not just a laughing matter. It's how they learn. Little ones are studying dozens of subjects simultaneously: how their bodies work, how they fit into their environments, how to communicate, what their limits are, and how to have fun. As with any new skill, when they're learning to play, babies need help. That's where you come in.

No matter what age your baby is, you'll keep his playtime fun by following certain general guidelines:

➤ Abandon the game after a couple of tries if the baby isn't interested or is balking.

➤ Don't pack his every waking minute with Creative Opportunities, Educational Experiences, and Fun-Fun-Fun. You're as likely to get agitation and tears as giggles. Babies need down time, too, and entertaining your little pashas every second of the day inhibits his natural ability to make his own fun.

➤ Respect the baby's time limits—little babies cannot sustain their focus for very long.

➤ Watch his response as you applaud his achievements. If he seems startled by your enthusiasm, tone it down a few notches.

➤ Help him along with a new game but don't *do* it for him. Let him try on his own. Let the victory be his.

➤ Keep in mind that babies are usually just as happy playing at home with you as they are with a trip to the circus.

➤ The best "toys" you can give your baby are your enthusiasm, your attention, and your joy.

➤ If you're having an off day, don't give yourself a hard time. A quiet afternoon together is itself a special sort of fun.

First Games for Newborns and Infants

Because your face and voice are so intriguing to the baby, give him plenty of opportunities to watch you and listen to you. Your lap is a perfect spot to play those first intimate games.

IN YOUR LAP

Prop your little one in your lap facing you and cradle his head in your hands. Then:

➤ Puff out your cheeks and press against them with the soles of the baby's feet; let the air rush out with a whoosh.

➤ Make faces by smiling, sticking out your tongue, blinking your eyes, wiggling your eyebrows.

➤ Chant, sing (see Chapter 6, "For a Song," and the "Words to Songs" appendix), hum, laugh, buzz, coo, whisper, babble, cluck, whistle, shush, click your tongue, or blow raspberries. Repeat the sounds the baby makes.

➤ Repeat a nonsense phrase such as "Biddy, biddy, biddy, boo." With each "biddy," move your face closer to his. At "boo," touch foreheads or touch noses.

➤ Speak in different tones (little ones show a marked preference for high-pitched voices).

➤ Gently shake your head and your hair.

➤ Let him hold your fingers. Wiggle them.

➤ Count his fingers and toes in a funny voice (see the "Words to Songs" appendix for games to play with fingers and toes).

➤ Clap his hands or feet or gently bicycle his legs.

➤ Provide counterpressure by letting him press his feet against your open hands.

➤ Dangle a bright-colored toy or shake a rattle for him to study.

➤ Let him "stand" or "hop" on your legs by supporting him under his arms (and along his neck if he can't support his head yet).

Keep games gentle, quiet, and brief.

GETTING DOWN ON ALL FLOORS

 Playing games with newborns on the floor requires only a clean, well-padded surface on which to play. Use a blanket, quilt, or beach towel. Here are some other ideas. Start with the baby lying on his back.

➤ Let him curl his fingers and toes around your finger.

➤ Massage him as you croon, "Mommy's rubbing your arm. Doesn't that feel nice?"

➤ Put bright-colored baby-size socks on his hands and watch his reaction. Some kids like this and some don't.

➤ Let him "track" (a fancy word for the baby's ability to follow something with his eyes) a bright toy, squeaky animal, or patterned object as you move it. Give him time to concentrate on one toy before exchanging it for another. Soon he'll try to grab it by bringing his hands together.

➤ Dangle a fabric ball, plastic doughnut, or soft toy on a ribbon and let him try to kick it.

➤ Lay him on his tummy and call his name or shake a rattle on either side of him. He'll turn his head to see what's going on and, eventually, start to raise his head and then push up, lifting head and chest clear of the floor.

➤ As he learns to push up while lying on his tummy, roll a bright-colored toy or chime ball within view. Before long, he'll be trying to scoot toward it.

T I P ➤ Experts warn against trying to influence a baby's development in a certain area, such as encouraging early dexterity in athletics or an appreciation for music. It's very premature. The skills your baby acquires in his first year happen naturally through his trial-and-error attempts. Simply provide a stimulating and nurturing environment in which he can develop and practice new skills. Keep things light and spontaneous.

BODY GAMES

With infants, keep physical activities short and take care not to overextend little limbs. Remember, this is not baby aerobics or a real workout. It's a game and the idea is to enjoy yourselves. Don't even think of starting an exercise regimen or gym class at this age. It's silly and potentially harmful. Instead, sing a song as you go (see Chapter 6, "For A Song," and the "Words to Songs" appendix) and proceed only if the baby is having a good time.

 To help him learn about his body, you can

➤ Lift his hands over his head and then down to his sides.

➤ Lift his hands outward from his body and back over his chest.

➤ Crisscross his arms over his chest slowly and rhythmically.

➤ Alternate arms, one up over the baby's head and the other down at his side.

➤ Hold the baby's ankles and push against one of his feet until his knee bends. Pull his foot back toward you, then switch to the other leg (we call this bicycling).

➤ Holding the baby's calves, straighten out his legs and then slowly push knees up to his chest and repeat. (This can help a baby pass gas, incidentally.)

You may have noticed your baby slowly blossoming from a tight newborn bud into an open flower. At first he seemed little more than a bundle of reflexes and responses, but now he is slowly emerging as an initiator of play. He will experiment with the ways in which his body and senses work and try, in his own clever ways (with eye contact, sounds, and body language), to let you know what he wants.

LIBBY: _I adored watching Sam "unfold" during his first weeks. He was like an underwater creature. His eyes blinked, his mouth worked in a dreamy kind of slow motion. His hands and fingers flexed and moved like a sea anemone being tugged by the tide. One of his favorite early games was to lie on the sofa and hypnotize himself with his hands._

Laughing It Up with a Lap Baby

No longer a dozy newborn, your baby is becoming more alert and has mastered several skills, such as visual tracking, pushing up with his arms when lying on his tummy, and grasping what he wants. Now the games you play will become a bit more sophisticated and a bit more exuberant.

PEEKABOO

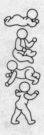

Peekaboo is magic. It has endless variations, requires no special equipment, works for little ones and toddlers, can be played with anyone, anywhere, anytime, and with anything. It rarely fails. When playing peekaboo, the baby is also exploring a very important concept known as object permanence: even though he can't see it, it's still there. Babies find this a reassuring, intriguing lesson and a wonderfully funny one, too.

To begin, hold your hands over your eyes and say, "Where did Daddy go?" or "Where's Mommy?" After a second or two, say, "Here's Daddy!" or "Here's Mommy!" Don't wait too long before you reappear, or you'll lose your audience to boredom or, worse, tears. (Use proper names, not pronouns, since little ones haven't conquered the use of I, he, she, and so on).

Change the tempo as you "reappear" gradually ("Heeeeeere's Kara") or add the element of surprise by holding on "peeeek-aaaaaa" and ending with an abrupt "boo." Don't scare him. If the whole process elicits a quivering bottom lip, stop.

Here are some variations of peekaboo that you can build on by adding your own twists:

➤ Cover the baby's eyes with your hands (or with a cloth diaper) for a split second and ask, "Where's baby?" and pull your hands away, "There he is!"

➤ Hold his hands over his eyes and then over your eyes.

➤ Hide behind a scarf, diaper, or blanket or peek around a large toy.

➤ Use a stuffed toy and hold its arms or paws over its eyes.

BABY'S BODY: INTRODUCING YOUR BABY TO HIS BODY

All babies need the time and the opportunity to figure out how their bodies work. Left to their own devices, babies will make these discoveries on their own. You don't want to squelch his desire to learn independently, but you can help his efforts along while you play.

➤ Encourage his efforts to practice stretching, head lifts, chest lifts, turning his head, inch-worming, and kicking by putting him first on his back, then, after a while, on his tummy.

➤ Let him practice his grip on your fingers. Don't try to put all of the baby's weight on his arms (he's probably not strong enough to support himself yet); just pull him toward you for a stretch and then let him pull his arms back.

➤ Sew a little bell securely onto the baby's sock. He'll soon start to kick his feet in order to hear it.

➤ Suspend a toy or ball (a beach ball works well) from a ribbon and dangle it over the baby as he's lying down. Instead of just gazing at it as he once did, he will bat at it with his hand or kick at it with his feet.

➤ Once he starts to practice rolling over, help him by giving him something to push off against, such as your hand.

➤ Let him "climb" up your chest as you hold him securely under his arms.

As your lap baby gains the muscle control that will enable him to sit, there are some entertaining activities for you to do together:

➤ Sit on the floor with the baby in your lap, his back nestled against your chest. Holding him securely, rock backward along your spine. The baby will love the ride.

➤ Sit down on the floor with your knees bent. Hold him so that his tummy is pressed against your shins. Roll onto your back and raise your legs and the baby. Bounce your legs as you hold his hands. Ride 'em, cowboy!

➤ Gently roll the baby, tummy down, over something cylindrical or spherical (like a beach ball). Don't let go for a second.

T I P ➤ If your baby is cranky and he's been in and out of his infant seat, car seat, stroller, or high chair all day, chances are he just needs some time to stretch out and relax. Place him on a brightly patterned blanket, quilt, or towel. If you've been in all day, he might crave a change of scene (don't you?). Try putting his infant seat or swing in a new position. Go for a walk.

Sitting Up and Taking Notice

Babies are dedicated scientists and avid explorers. As your baby becomes more at ease with his body, he'll also begin to understand the world around him. One way that he'll achieve this is through experimenting with simple cause-and-effect relationships.

FILL 'ER UP AND TIP 'EM OUT

Babies love the repetitive nature of filling up containers and dumping out the contents. The basic way to set up the game is to give your baby two unbreakable containers (clean plastic yogurt or margarine containers do nicely). Put some smaller objects inside (make sure they're too big to swallow) and show him how to move them by hand from one container to another. Once he masters that, you can show him how to pour them back and forth.

There are all kinds of ways to vary this game, such as exaggerating the size and shape of the containers and the objects. You can try leaving the lid on the container to see if his tiny fingers can remove it and put it back on. You can use transparent containers or opaque ones. You can play it in the kitchen with measuring spoons, in the bath with plastic toys, or in the backyard with clothespins. You can pour a teeny bit of water into the container.

T I P ➤ You may notice periodically during your baby's first year that he spends much of his day doing one thing over and over again. Don't discourage him or distract him with something else unless he seems frustrated. He's not bored. He's happy. He's also developing his powers of concentration, his manual dexterity, and probably a bunch of other skills the pediatricians haven't told us about yet.

He will invent many of his own cause-and-effect games, but here are some you can introduce:

➤ Repeat his words back to him ("Mama hears George say ba ba ba ba"), and he will enthusiastically try to respond to you.

➤ Lightly touch one of the baby's features (noses work well), making a sound. When the baby touches your nose, make the sound.

➤ Show him how to use a toy that rattles, chimes, or squeaks.

➤ Let him turn the light switch off and on.

➤ Blow bubbles and pop them with his finger.

➤ Churn or splash his hands and feet in the tub.

➤ Stack nesting cups or blocks and knock them over with his hand.

➤ Look through a pop-up book or fiddle with an activity center.

To make peekaboo games a little more challenging:

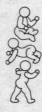

➤ Place a cloth diaper or scarf over a rattle or other toy. Ask, "Where did the rattle go?" At first, you uncover it with an enthusiastic "There it is!" Next time, leave a little edge sticking out. Soon he'll jubilantly uncover the toy himself.

➤ Place a cloth diaper over his foot or hand. "Where did Sam's hand go?" This helps him learn the words for the parts of his body, too.

➤ Sink below view (below the crib bumpers or behind the sofa) and ask, "Where's Daddy?" Then pop up at a different spot.

➤ Play hide-and-seek by "hiding" a toy in your hand, in a pocket, or under your (or the baby's) shirt and let him find it.

LOIS: *One day when Annie was five months old, as I was changing her, she pulled a cloth diaper over her face. As I reached for the wipes, I said, "Where's Annie?" hoping that she wasn't frightened under the diaper and unable to pull it away. Silly me. She pulled it off, laughed, and then put it back over her face as if to say, "Come on. Get with it."*

ANKLES AWAY: BOUNCING GAMES FOR SITTING BABIES

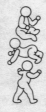

A sturdily sitting baby is ready for any of the traditional games in which the baby sits on your lap or straddles your foot (and holds on to your leg for dear life) while you bounce him up and down and repeat a rhyme. Part of his pleasure is at having your full attention, and part of it is the thrill of ending the game with an especially vigorous bounce and, perhaps, sinking between your knees. (Whoa, cowboy! Don't try these games right after a feeding.)

LAURIE: *Anna always enjoyed bouncing on my knee to "Humpty Dumpty." When he had his great fall, she'd slip between my knees and guffaw. Then she'd bounce for more.*

Start bouncing games sedately and build to the level of raucousness your baby likes. Just be sure you are holding him comfortably and securely and that he's well-balanced. Some of the ditties will transport you back to your own childhood; "Ride a Cock Horse" has been around for generations:

> Ride a cock horse to Banbury Cross,
> To see a fine lady upon a white horse.
> With rings on her fingers and bells on her toes,
> She shall have music wherever she goes.

Lyrics to some of our other favorites are listed in the "Words to Songs" appendix. When words escape you, there's always "three, two, one, blast-off" to transport your little astronaut to giggle heaven.

_____

T I P ➤ It's worth borrowing a copy of *Music for Very Little People: 50 Playful Activities for Infants and Toddlers* (John M. Feierabend, Farmingdale, N.Y.: Boosey & Hawkes, Inc., 1986) from your library. It's a tape on which practically every little ditty is sung or recited, and they're all grouped by activity: bounces, wiggles, tickles, tapping, clapping, circles, and lullabies.

_____

HEDY: *When Molly rides on my ankle, we sing "Huppa, Huppa Rida," a German nursery rhyme. Although my father is German, I hadn't cared to learn much of the language before Molly was born; but I really wanted to be able to sing the same song to her that my grandmother had sung to my father and my father had sung to me.*

If you think back (or call home), you're sure to rediscover other little games your grandmother taught your mother and your mother taught you. Completing this circle, you may want to pass on these amusements to your babe.

GENNY: *When Kara was five months old, my mom visited and played chin chopper with her (see the "Words to Songs" appendix). The next time they saw each other, months later, Kara's first words were "chin chopper."*

All games like these help the baby learn to communicate at the same time as they enhance his motor coordination. Of course, you'll have to guide the baby's movements at first. Other baby classics include:

➤ clapping hands

➤ shaking his head no and nodding yes

➤ waving hello and bye-bye

➤ blowing kisses

➤ slapping high and low fives (a contemporary classic)

➤ putting both arms over his head to make the touchdown signal

➤ so big

Pat-a-cake is another universal hit. Since clapping hands is a skill babies learn fairly early on, starting around seven months, it's one of the first true games they can learn. It's also a game babies soon discover they have in common with others in their social set.

Here are the words to this classic (there are other versions), along with the hand motions:

Pat-a-cake *(clap)*
Pat-a-cake *(clap)*
Baker's man *(clap)*.
Bake me *(clap)* a cake *(clap)* as fast *(clap)* as you can *(clap)*.
Pat it *(make patting motions)*, and prick it *(poke baby's tummy)*,
And mark it with a "B" *(draw letter on baby's tummy)*.
And put it in the oven *(slide your hands toward baby and tickle him)*
For baby *(point to him)* and me *(point to yourself)*.

The trick here is to recite the rhyme with gusto as you clap the baby's hands together. Make it seem suspenseful—like an exciting story with a fascinating ending. In the beginning, consistent repetition works best. As your baby catches on, you can put a new spin on it:

➤ Invent new words for the last two lines so that they rhyme with the baby's own initial, or substitute other familiar names, as in, "Put it in the oven for Pop-Pop and me."

➤ Clap feet inside of hands.

➤ Change "cake," to "banana" or "pretzel" or something else edible with which your baby is familiar.

➤ Make up new words such as, "Fill it with lemon and mix it with spice and serve it to my baby with everything nice."

➤ Tickle the baby when you draw the "B".

LIVELIER GAMES FOR SITTING BABIES

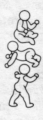 As your baby becomes more adept at getting into a sitting position, there are other kinds of physical games the two of you can try out. Do keep in mind that little bodies are fragile bodies and that every child has his own preference about how rough he likes to play. More physical games you can try with your baby are:

➤ Sit on the floor with your knees bent, sit the baby on top of your knees, hold his hands, and slide him down till he's sitting on your tummy. Or slide him from your knees down to your toes. It's more comfortable if you lean against the sofa or a wall.

➤ Lie down on your back. Sit the baby on your stomach with his legs straddling you. Hold onto his hands as you lift your hips slightly. Sing the theme to "Rawhide" if the spirit moves you.

➤ Give him a modified piggy back ride: wrap his arms around your neck and hold his hands with one of your own. Bring your other arm around your back and support his bottom.

➤ Let him ride on your shoulders with his legs around your neck, your fingers laced together supporting his back. Be prepared for him to rest his head on yours and to pull your hair. Obviously, watch out for low clearances.

➤ Hold him around his upper chest and swing him back and forth between your legs. *Never* swing a child of any age by his arms alone; dislocated shoulders happen all too often.

➤ Play roller baby: lie down on your back and lie him face down on your chest. Wrap your arms around him and roll first to one side, then back to the middle, and then over to the other side and back to the middle.

➤ Go flying. Hold the baby securely around his chest and fly him around like a jet. Make whatever aerodynamic noises you can. One friend used to pretend that Molly was a fighter plane and made shooting noises as he flew her around. She liked it.

JIL: *"Flying" has always been one of Jenny's favorite activities. Zooming into people's faces and startling them was especially funny to her. "Let's fly to Jenny's room" was a happy distraction that stilled many tears of frustration when we had to remove her from something dangerous that had caught her attention.*

➤ Create a major distraction. Molly's dad jokingly called it "changing the baby's reality." Pick the baby up, hold him securely to your chest, make a funny noise, and spin quickly around a couple of times. Or, run as fast as you can for a short distance. Through his giggles, the baby no longer cares that he was crying a second ago.

As you enjoy a hearty play period together, watch for the baby's signals that he's tiring: he may divert his eyes or rub them, fret, or crawl away. He's disengaging, giving you a message to start the settling-down ritual. Wind down by lying together quietly. Offer him a drink and a snack. This helps your baby get used to the rhythm of life and keeps him from becoming too rambunctious for too long, which leads very quickly to tension and tears.

HAVE A BALL!

Like plastic cups, balls are way up there on our versatility list. And they are many babies' favorite first toys. They can be thrown, caught, kicked, batted, bounced, and best of all, chased (on hands and knees). There are lots of different kinds, each with a characteristic to recommend it (choose balls larger than two inches in diameter to prevent choking accidents, and remember, they'll also get chewed—so no sponge balls or balls that can have pieces bitten off):

➤ Soft multicolored fabric balls are fun for lap and sitting babies to study.

➤ There are weighted balls that don't roll out of reach, a frequent frustration to precrawlers. (Small beanbags don't roll away either and are easy for babies to grab; they can be used as substitutes in some ball games, as can cylinders).

➤ Beautiful, hand-crafted, textured fabric balls are designed for pick-up-ability.

➤ The movement of a ball within a ball entrances babies; the sound of a chime within a ball delights them.

➤ An inflatable ball makes a great park or travel toy since you can just let the air out when you're done to fit it in a stroller bag.

Here are some ball games for babies who can sit up by themselves (spread their legs slightly to play):

➤ Roll a ball to him. He won't even consider rolling it back. But he'll like seeing it come toward him and finding it within reach.

➤ Sit him at the bottom of a ramp or slide and roll a ball down to him. Or roll it through a tube or under a bridge (made with blocks or books or in a playground).

➤ Give a ball to the baby when he's in his playpen or other confined area. That way, he can retrieve it when it rolls away.

➤ Go bowling by setting up a couple of easy-to-knock-down blocks, and guide the baby's hand as he rolls the ball for a strike.

➤ Play soccer by holding the baby around his ribs and supporting his bottom and gently swinging him so that his feet kick the ball.

➤ Bring a plastic ball into the bathtub, put the baby's hand on it, put your own hand on top of his, and hold the ball under water. Let go and watch the surprise on his face as the ball pops up to the surface. Oooh, physics.

PAULA: *Toward the end of his first year, George developed a grand ball obsession. We couldn't pass a store with a ball in the window without him straining to get out of his stroller to go inside. He didn't even realize he couldn't walk yet. I considered putting a limit on the number of balls I'd buy but then I realized that balls are cheap and don't cause cavities. So I bought him a lot of balls.*

KNOCKING BLOCKS

The simplest block building (see Chapter 5, "Toy with Me," for product recommendations) will delight a baby this age: build a tower and show him how to knock it over. To add variety:

➤ Show him (using rectangular blocks) how the domino effect works.

➤ Make a roadway for cars, a maze, or a ramp for balls.

➤ Make a castle for his toy cars and dolls.

➤ Make geometric designs or pictures.

➤ Count the blocks or name the colors as you build.

➤ Arrange blocks by color and shapes as you say, "One red circle, one blue square."

TRICKS OF THE BABY TRADE

If you catch a certain expression or funny habit your baby is experimenting with and repeating, give it a name. He will soon be able to "perform" it, usually happily, whenever you prompt him. Most of our kids had one or two quirky mannerisms that we named and encouraged; a couple weren't into it at all. If it's a trick you'd just as soon he forgot, don't name it and don't laugh at it or otherwise call attention to it. Without encouragement, he may never repeat it.

Yes, we know. Children are not trained seals to perform on command for a kipper snack. But check out the look on your baby's face when he's done his little act and everyone around him claps and grins. Most babies are hams, so don't deny yourself (or your little grandstander) the fun. Of course, don't badger your "star" if he's not yearning for the spotlight or if he just plain doesn't enjoy the attention.

LAURIE: *Anna loved getting into the act. One of her favorite performance pieces was "Tick Tock." I'd hold her around her waist, pick her up, and swing her from side to side while singing, "Tick tock, tick tock. I'm a little cuckoo clock. Now I'm striking two o'clock!" then swing her up and out for the "cuckoo cuckoo" part.*

Here are some "tricks" our kids learned before their first birthdays:

➤ "Where's the blackbird?" Your baby points skyward and gets tickled under his arm.

➤ The "Claus von Bulow" look, Anna's formidable scowl.

➤ "Fish face," Molly's way of sucking in her cheeks.

➤ "Bat face," Annie's Bela Lugosi-ish way of showing her first two teeth—her lateral incisors.

➤ "Sweet Eyes," Sam and Molly's way of blinking rapidly to simulate a flirtatious look.

➤ "Sing Hallelujah." Annie would raise her arms over her head and waggle both her hands at the wrist.

SHADOW PLAY

One day, somewhere between six and eight months, your baby may notice shadows. Like most everything else, however, he'll discover this little wonder sooner with your help.

Begin by showing him his shadow, yours, his stroller's, the dog's. Watch for interesting shadows and point them out when you spot them. If your child is intrigued, you may want to learn to make shadows with your hands. You'll dazzle your baby and his friends. Later, add balloon animals, magic tricks, juggling, or face painting, and you'll have nifty skills to offer when it comes time to volunteer at preschool functions.

T I P ➤ If you want to make soaring eagles, hopping bunnies, and barking dogs on the wall by lamplight, there are books on the subject. Two are: *The Little Book of Shadows* by Phila H. Webb and Jane Gerby (Philadelphia: Running Press, 1990) and *Shadows Are About* by Ann Whitford Paul (New york: Scholastic, Inc., 1992). These make great Father's and Mother's Day gifts.

Crawling Toward Home

Now that your baby is crawling, it's time for you to hit the floor, too. Crawl down the hall, around the chair, and under the table with your little explorer. It's wonderful fun (albeit hard on the knees), and your company is guaranteed to delight your baby. You're also bound to find the baby's-eye view enlightening (go on a safety hunt while you're down there and check for socket covers and such).

SIMPLE GAMES FOR CRAWLERS

Active frolicking will please him most at this stage. Peekaboo games in which he has to move or do something to find the object are popular, too:

➤ Sam and Molly gleefully played tag on their hands and knees around and around a room divider. Libby or Hedy had to instigate the game initially, of course, but the babies soon learned to get started on their own.

➤ Annie liked leading crawling parades with Mommy, Daddy, and Blazer (the dog), in that order, please, in tow.

➤ Hide a musical toy in another room and send him to find it.

➤ Hide a toy under one of three cups, shuffle them around, and let him try to find it.

➤ When his hand is out of view (say, under the tray of his high chair), ask, "Where did George's hand go?" (look really perplexed). When he whips it back into view, say, "There it is!"

➤ Bury a sand toy in view but out of reach in the sandbox under an obvious mound.

➤ Play the nose-chin game (one of Chuck and Sam's first games): have the baby press the tip of your nose. When he does, stick your tongue out. Have him press your chin, and bring your tongue back in. Later on you can teach him to tug one ear to have your tongue move one way, the other ear to have it go the other way.

APPEALING TO HIS SENSES

Now that your baby has developed more of an attention span, there are even more games that help him learn about the world. His senses are becoming more sophisticated, and there are plenty of sensory games to play:

➤ Start his exploration of smell with the obvious—flowers. Let him watch as you sniff a flower and then give him a turn with something really fragrant, such as roses, honeysuckle, or freesia. Take him to the local florist for a real noseful.

➤ Introduce him to various pleasant-smelling things such as shampoo, a fresh-cut orange, or fresh bread. (Remember that a baby's sense of smell is much more acute than an adult's, so be judicious.)

➤ School his ears by stopping whatever you're doing when you hear a sound (the doorbell, the timer on the microwave, Daddy opening the Doritos, the dog barking). Ask the baby, "What is making that sound?" Find the source together.

➤ Give him a selection of "drums and drumsticks"—cardboard containers, metal mixing bowls, plastic flowerpots, rubber spatulas, wooden spoons—so he can experiment with different sound combinations.

➤ Use hand signals and explanatory gestures when asking him to do something or making conversation so he'll start to associate visual cues with auditory ones.

➤ Describe things by their colors, shapes, and other identifying marks so he starts to understand what differentiates one thing from another.

➤ Let him learn about the variety of textures in the world by giving him a piece of corduroy to play with. As he touches it, say "bumpy" over and over; say "smooth" with a piece of satin; "wet" with water; and so on.

➤ Start teaching him the subtle variations of touch by working on "gentle" (see Animal Magnetism in Chapter 2, "Domestic Bliss"). Early on, you can help him understand that he has control of his hands by practicing with him on a fluffly stuffed animal. Then let him loose on your neighbor's (declawed) cat.

Cruisin'

Cruisers are amazing creatures. Holding on, they "walk" and they "talk." Their hands are otherwise occupied, but their gums, they are aflapping. Here are some games for this exciting time.

THE NAME GAME

This is a time when many babies start to show a growing interest in words and names for things. To enhance his natural desire (no flash cards, please) to understand language:

➤ Put several different toys in a box. Ask for one by its name. When the baby gives you a blank stare, pick up the toy and say, "Here's the mouse." Put it back and ask again. Soon he'll be handing you Mickey himself, even when you ask for the rattle.

➤ Play with puppets, using a crib or playpen for a theater, to tell simple stories using the words he is learning. Be careful here: puppets frighten some babies.

➤ Feed Teddy, comb Teddy's fur, rock Teddy, kiss Teddy, wave bye-bye to Teddy, making sure that you are clearly naming each activity.

➤ Name the baby's body parts (in the bath, while getting changed, and so on). It's a valuable lesson especially as you go about teaching other new skills (get your foot off the kitty's foot).

➤ When you come across a word in a song or book that you can point out in the baby's environment, show it to him right then. This is how your baby will learn vocabulary.

FUN WITH FIRST WORDS

An entertaining way to introduce some first words is to use opposites. For instance: In a loud voice say, "LOUD LOUD LOUD" and then in a whisper say, "quiet quiet quiet." Repeat it several times. No matter what the word is, always use a toy, your bodies, or some other method of clearly demonstrating the difference. Other word combinations that work well are:

- Push-Pull
- Up-Down
- Bumpy-Smooth
- Happy-Sad
- Big-Little
- Front-Back
- Open-Closed

- Fast-Slow
- Over-Under
- On-Off
- High-Low
- Bye-Bye–Hello
- Go-Stop
- Soft-Hard

THAT'S SILLY

 As babies begin to understand rules, order, simple physical laws, what's what, and who's who, they also begin to appreciate incongruities. In fact, babies adore incongruities. When something is presented to them that is backward, upside-down, or ridiculous, they are struck by the silliness of it and get the joke.

LOIS: *One day when Annie was about seven months old, I stuck one of her pink socks on our dog's head. Blazer cocked her head, looking very much like the RCA dog in a tiny pink beret, and Annie let out a big hardee-har-har.*

To open a window on your little one's budding sense of humor, here are some other "what's funny about this picture" scenarios you can stage:

➤ Put a diaper on a panda or give a bottle to a truck as you feign total seriousness.

➤ Put something of the baby's on you (a bib or his shoe).

➤ Pretend to climb into his high chair or tell another grownup that it's time to go in the stroller for a walk.

➤ Crawl around on the floor mimicking the family pet.

➤ Use a toy telephone as if it were the real thing. Then hand it to him, saying, "It's for you."

Be as goofy as your imagination (and self-respect) allow. Remember, it's worth being silly to hear that delicious giggle.

PLAY BALL!

 When your cruiser is ready for a game that doesn't require your holding his hands so he can walk to Timbuktu and back, play ball. Now that his hand-eye coordination is better developed, the ball games you can play together can be more interactive.

➤ Roll balls of various sizes between you. Roll more than one at a time. Roll one to him as he rolls one to you.

➤ Roll a ball under something else (a table), and ask, "Where did George's ball go? *There* it is!" He might even want to crawl over and get it himself.

➤ See if he can roll a ball into a bucket (make it easy by using a large bucket).

➤ If he can stand on his own two feet, take batting practice by giving him a toy broom or rolling a ball at him and letting him swat at it. Guide him so he actually hits it once in a while or he'll lose interest.

GAMES WE DISCOURAGED

 For one reason or another, there were certain games that some or all of us did not encourage our kids to play. These include:

➤ Tearing up newspapers, magazines, or other printed material. Some inks are toxic. Also, a baby cannot differentiate between junk mail, the photographs you cherish, and first editions.

➤ Bathtub crayons: "Since I'm allowed to write on the bathtub wall with crayons," the baby thinks, "why don't I write on the living room wall, too?"

➤ Bath books: your baby may decide to lob all printed material into the tub or toilet when your back is turned.

➤ Throwing: we all agreed early on that only balls and kisses are for throwing.

You're ready to have a jolly old time? Great. The keys are simple: Match games to your child's ability and mood. Be creative and take advantage of whatever's around you. Leave time for a cool-down period after exuberant playtime. And be prepared to perform on command once your baby discovers what a clever, fun-loving parent you are.

5

TOY WITH ME

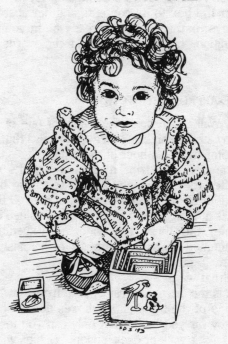

Although it may look like a day at the beach, a baby's life is no picnic. From the moment they are born, babies are on the job. Play is a baby's work and toys are her tools. Your job is to make sure her workplace is safe, to stock it with the materials she needs, and to provide a generous vacation package.

Toys help your baby experiment, explore, and, eventually, manipulate her environment. They help her develop physical prowess and expand her intellectual, emotional, social, and creative capacities. And if those developmental issues weren't enough, think about what fun you're going to have playing with toys you enjoyed as a kid. The classics are back.

Toys! What to Know Before You Choose

Webster's says that a toy is "something for a child to play with." You can buy them, be them, improvise them, or make them yourself. But don't spend your life savings on toys. Your little one will often prefer the box to its contents and her absolute favorite toy (a set of keys, perhaps) might already be in your pocket. To Webster's definition, however, we'd add the words "safe" and "appropriate."

SELECTING AGE-APPROPRIATE TOYS

 Walking through the aisles of one of those large toy stores can bring on a queasiness that can only be compared to a bout of morning sickness. It's one of the first field trips most new parents make, right after they've opened all the receiving blankets and adorable outfits and thought, in panic, "But the baby has nothing to play with." Our combined experiences with the First Toy Shopping Expedition can be summed up as a synthesis of astonishment, awe, dread, guilt, and intimidation.

It needn't be that way.

The problem is the dizzying array of stuff from which to choose. The bullying tone of the hype on the boxes doesn't help: "If you don't buy this toy for your child, not only can you forget college, she may never talk or walk or use a spoon!" Babies will learn basic skills with "educational" toys or without them, for fun is the most powerful developmental aid on the market, and you, dear parent, are the Master of Amusement.

And what about those little age groupings in the corner of the box? Will you be keeping your three-month-old back if you buy her a rattle marked "birth to six months"? Will she have a better chance of becoming a brain surgeon if you get her the firehouse marked "one year and up"? Should you take out a second mortgage and buy one of everything?

Don't go bananas in front of Curious George. Basically, if you can answer yes to these six questions while holding the toy, it's probably a good buy:

➤ Is it "developmentally correct" (will she be able to use it) or educational (will she learn something new from it)?

➤ Will it stimulate her?

➤ Is it fun?

➤ Can it be used in more than one way?

➤ Does it look as if it will last?

➤ Can you afford it?

The age-range labels on boxes follow U.S. Consumer Product Safety Commission guidelines, which are based on a child's physical and mental capacities to understand and manipulate a toy; developmental needs and interests; and the safety of the toy for each age level. Many labels say only that the toy is not for children under three, usually because of small, swallowable parts. If the age range on a toy seems absurdly long to you (say, "six months to five years"), it's probably an attempt on the toy maker's part to boost sales.

As for whether the toy will stimulate _your_ baby, only you know what captivates her and how quickly she is developing. For every child who loved her xylophone at nine months, there's another who showed no interest until she was two. In order to formulate an educated guess, notice which toys your baby already likes to play with, watch which toys interest your baby at the pediatrician's office, at day care, and at other people's homes, and see what she is drawn to first.

Is your baby going to have fun with this toy? Again, go by the best acid test you have: your knowledge of your child. Is she a shaker or a mouther? Does she like hugging furry bears or throwing balls? Is she a more active babe who likes things that move, or a contemplative type, content to stare at an intricate pattern for hours?

JIL: _When Jenny was three and a half months old, she made her first toy selection. I carried her around the store picking things off the shelf from time to time and showing them to her. She reached for a multicolored ball, mouthed it, and would not let it go. I was drawn to another, more expensive toy. We bought both. I have no idea what happened to my choice, but we still play with the ball._

Two toy-buying caveats: 1) A toy that is too difficult for the child may undermine her budding self-confidence, and she won't continue to play with it. 2) There is no "right" way to play with a toy. Your baby will find uses for toys that neither you nor the manufacturer would have imagined. Still, if a toy comes with instructions or play suggestions, read them; *you* might learn something.

LIBBY: *Sam had a peg board meant to help him explore patterns and colors while refining his fine-motor coordination. The instructions all but promised he'd be flying a jet within the year. Sam used the pegs as passengers in his little cars and liked to roll them at dust balls under the furniture.*

Can you do lots of different things with the toy? Can you build different games around it? Can it go into the bath? Will it be fun to play with outside? Is it a good traveling toy? Certainly, no toy can be all things to all babies, but versatility promotes creative play (mainly on your part at this age) and extends the "life" of the toy.

Will the toy withstand teething, throwing, being run over by a stroller, and other predictably unorthodox uses? Is it washable or can you otherwise clean it? If a toy is going to get too grubby too soon, wear out, or fall apart from use, it's not worth the money.

Before you head for the store, quiz your friends with little ones about their children's tried-and-trues. Write down brand names and, especially if you're looking for a particular toy, call ahead; some large chains only carry certain brands. Read the articles about toys, toy ratings, and toy selection in parenting magazines. Such toy roundups are usually published in November and December issues in time for holiday gift buying. Look carefully at illustrations or photographs of toys in advertisements. Also consult *Consumer Reports*.

Many toy manufacturers will send catalogues of their products so you can review what's available before you go shopping:

➤ Fisher Price: (800) 432-5437

➤ Little Tikes: (800) 321-0183

➤ Mattel: (800) 421-2887

➤ Playskool: (800) PLAYSKL

There are also several books on the toy topic:

The Childwise Catalog: A Consumer Guide to Buying the Safest and Best Products for Your Children by Jack Gillis and Mary Ellen R. Fise (New York: Perennial Library, 1990).

The Kids' Catalog Collection: A Selective Guide to More than 500 Catalogs Jam-packed with Toys, Books, Clothes, Sporting Goods, Party Supplies and Everything Else Kids Want and Need by Jane Smolnik (Chester, Conn.: The Globe Pequot Press, 1990).

Smart Toys by Kent Garland Burtt and Karen Kalstein (New York: Harper & Row, 1981).

Making Your Own Toys by Pamela Peake (Emmaus, Penn.: Rodale Press, 1986).

FOR SAFEKEEPING

There are governmental agencies that monitor toy safety, but some people question whether federal standards, or the toy manufacturers' compliance with them, are adequate. You should be able to answer yes to all the toy safety questions in this checklist while satisfying your own instincts. If a sample of the toy isn't on display, ask for one; you may have to insist or see a manager.

➤ Is every part of the toy too big to fit completely into the baby's mouth? (The No-Choke Testing Tube, a device that gauges small toy parts to see whether an infant or toddler could choke on them, is available for $1.00 from Toys to Grow On, Box 17, Long Beach, CA 90801; (800) 542-8338.)

➤ Are all the parts, decorations, and features (eyes, noses, buttons, and such) fastened securely so they can't be pulled or bitten off? Is the toy free of strings or ribbons?

➤ Are all the edges rounded and smooth?

➤ Does the toy seem sturdy and unbreakable? Are the seams sealed properly? Does the fur stay attached if you gently tug at it? If it has a liquid element, is it well encased?

➤ Is the toy made and decorated with nontoxic materials?

➤ On hand-crafted wooden toys, does the paint chip easily or the wood splinter?

➤ Is the toy made in the United States? Toy manufacturers in foreign countries may not have to follow domestic standards. Check foreign-made toys extra carefully before buying.

Remember that *all* toys for kids one and under require appropriate adult supervision. And if you have older kids or visit someone who does, be careful to keep their more sophisticated toys out of reach.

There are various publications on toy safety available:

➤ "Which Toy for Which Child," a pair of booklets (one covers infants through age five, the other six through twelve) from the Federal Consumer Safety Commission, Washington, DC 20207.

➤ "The T.M.A. Guide to Toys and Play," Toy Manufacturers of America, Box 866, Madison Square Station, New York, NY 10159.

➤ "Be Sure It's Safe for Your Baby," Juvenile Products Manufacturers Association, 2 Greentree Center, Suite 225, Marlton, NJ 08053.

➤ "The 1991 Toy Safety Report," Institute for Injury Reduction, Box 1621, Upper Marlboro, MD 20772; $1.

➤ "Trouble in Toyland," United States Public Interest Research Group, 215 Pennsylvania Ave. SE, Washington, DC 20003; $6.

GOING FOR BROKE: SHOPPING WELL AND BUYING RIGHT

When you venture out for toys for the first time, memorize the toy-shopping mantra:

➤ There is no such thing as one perfect toy that will make my baby smarter or happier than she already is.

➤ There is no such thing as an essential toy that my baby must have in order to thrive.

➤ More expensive is not necessarily better.

➤ My baby doesn't need (and shouldn't have) every toy on the market.

Then, go shop. Start at a smaller toy store or a five-and-dime. Whereas the chains offer discounts, selection, specials, and coupons, those massive hangars can be just too much for your first expeditions. It's easy to overspend. Once you have an idea of what's out there and what you want (and your postpartum hormonal storms—if you're having them—have subsided), head for the big stores.

LIBBY: _When Sam was six months old, all three of us went on an expedition to a BIG toy store. In minutes, I'd filled the cart as if it were Giveaway Day. Chuck deprogrammed me with a stern "get ahold of yourself" chat. We ended up with three toys we knew from our past and from the pediatrician's office: a shape sorter, a chime ball, and an activity box. It was plenty._

Our shopping tips are:

➤ When you can, shop with your child so you can test the toy out on her. Bribe another adult to come along so that one of you can take care of baby and the other the business at hand. Going with another parent and child is also an option; the adults alternate shopping and caring for the youngsters.

➤ Save receipts and boxes for a while after you open the toy. It's easy to lose track of what you already have, and the baby might not show an interest in what you've chosen. Don't be hurt, and get used to it. If you love the toy and suspect that the baby's lack of interest is simply that she's not ready for it, put it away for a while and reintroduce it later.

➤ Borrow big-ticket toys from friends or relatives before you buy them. This is not foolproof, however. We've seen it dozens of times: Kara is entranced by George's new Big Bird activity center, so Genny surprises Kara with one, and Kara never touches it. A toy's cachet is often that it's at someone else's house.

➤ Even if you've come home with a dozen new toys, don't unpack them all right away. The baby can only deal with one new toy at a time. Keep this advice in mind at holiday and first-birthday time (see the appendix "A Word on First Birthdays"), when your baby gets to know the UPS delivery person on a first-name basis.

Ballooning Responsibility

Inflated balloons are fun. They're colorful, light, cheerful, versatile, and cheap. Yet an uninflated balloon or a piece of a popped balloon can choke or suffocate a child. *Always* supervise balloon play with children. *Never* let a child put a balloon near her mouth. Better substitutes are Mylar balloons, punch balls, or beach balls. They are much harder to pop, bite, or break, and they stay inflated longer. Discard balloons before they begin to deflate or are lost under the bed. If you see a popped balloon on the ground, pick up the pieces and throw them away.

You needn't think of toy stores as your only shopping source. You can pick up a bonanza of second-hand toys at school fairs, yard sales, and consignment shops. Check the bulletin board at your pediatrician's office. Mail-order catalogues are another source. The following ones specialize in toys (see the "Mail Order Sources" appendix for addresses):

- HearthSong
- Childcraft
- The Great Kids Co.
- Toys to Grow On
- F. A. O. Schwarz
- Back to Basics Toys
- Lillian Vernon
- Sesame Street Catalog
- Animal Town
- Just for Kids!
- Sensational Beginnings

Museum catalogues often feature unusual toys, too.

Parents magazine has a kind of toy club for newborns through preschoolers. They bought out Johnson & Johnson's toy catalogue program and feature the Johnson & Johnson toys (Wiggle Worm, Red Rings, and others). Every four to six weeks, subscribers receive by mail a toy or two designed to coincide with your baby's advancing developmental stages. Each toy comes with a booklet describing different games and ways to play. The toys are well conceived, well-made, and popular with little ones. For information, call (800) 678-2686.

Another option is Discovery Toys. These toys are sold through local representatives and get-togethers (like Tupperware). For more information call (800) 426-4777.

First Toys for Newborns

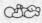 What? You mean the kid's got to have something as soon as she hits the air? Next thing you know some genius will be marketing toys for the womb.

LAURIE: *Before Anna's birth we were given a black-and-white elephant. The label directed us to give it to our baby on day one. We dutifully placed Mr. Elephant in Anna's hospital nursery bassinet. Anna immediately sat up and started talking to it in complete sentences. Truth be told, she paid no attention to poor Mr. E. at all.*

All toys (except you) are pretty superfluous in the first few weeks of life. Your newborn has enough to do acclimating to her new environment. She won't even be able to voluntarily uncurl her fingers to hold onto an object for several weeks. During this adjustment period, her (and your) day will pretty much be taken up with eating and sleeping. She'll consider her fingers, fist, pacifier, and anything on which she can suck fine "toys."

 Toward the end of the first month, babies start to show growing interest in the external world. Throughout this time, as we have said, her first "toy" will be you—your fingers, your voice, your smell, your facial expressions. When she is able to focus on objects that are farther away, she'll love looking at faces—human and toy. And, she'll notice, focus on, and pay attention to her surroundings more.

 In the first three months of life, recent research tells us, a baby sees high-contrast, black-and-white, geometric designs best. Manufacturers of all sorts of baby equipment have jumped on this bandwagon and produced everything from mobiles to crib linens in black and white.

Most of the newborns we know did indeed seem to focus on black-and-white patterns. But there's no need to create a baby disco. We found black and white great for mobiles and a few other items, including those little stuffed critters around week four.

If you make sure that all toys can be safely gummed, rolled on, or tipped onto her, playthings that will amuse her include:

➤ A vinyl accordion-style foldout book with any combination of an unbreakable plastic mirror, faces, checkerboards, bull's-eyes, and other geometric designs. The *Let's Look Book* (Discovery Toys, 2530 Arnold Dr., Suite 400, Martinez, CA 94453 [1987] (800) 426-4777) gets points for versatility because one side has black-and-white geometric patterns, which will appeal to your baby now, and the other shows faces, which will fascinate your baby in a few weeks. Made of vinyl, it can be propped up easily in a crib or playpen, on a changing table, or in a car. And it's chewable.

➤ Soft, lightweight rattles. One that you fasten to the baby's wrist with Velcro can be fun; just make sure to remove it when the baby's amusement wanes.

➤ Small, textured balls that she can grasp and wave; if there's a bell inside, she'll like it even more.

➤ Little creatures with simple faces may appeal to her; the ones made of vinyl, rubber, or terry cloth are best for mouthing.

You'll find yourself awash with stuffed animals and dolls without ever purchasing a single one yourself; people love giving them as gifts. Most babies show as much interest in stuffed animals as they do in the stock market. For the time being, pile them on shelves and use them to make the nursery look ever so *baby*. Don't despair. In eighteen months or so, their day will come.

Lap Baby Toys

 By about the fourth month a baby will be drawn to bright colors. She's going to start really responding to faces. A soft rattle in the shape of an animal or a little stuffed creature with a simple face will delight her. Many babies take to Mickey or Minnie Mouse around this time in a big way. But she won't have any clue about toys unless you introduce them to her.

LIBBY: *In Sam's first months, he seemed so fragile. I fretted he might bean his fontanelle with his plastic duck or be scared silly by the musical pillow. Sam's first sitter, Li Li, taught Sam at four months to grasp the noisiest rattle and shake it for all he was worth. For him, no bell was too loud, no squeaker too startling.*

Although lap babies still need you to support their seemingly boneless little bodies, they are beginning to swat their arms and kick those pudgy legs with excitement. New toys that take advantage of these newfound abilities are:

➤ Crib gyms: these are toys meant for suspending over cribs. They look a lot like outdoor swing sets except that the dangling parts are mirrors, chimes, faces, and sparkly bits, often decorated with Disney or "Sesame Street" characters. They help babies experiment with their ever-improving muscle control. Remove these gyms when the baby is able to pull herself up. There are freestanding A-frame versions with things to whirl, spin, and jangle, all meant for floor play. (Some of our kids found these too stimulating at first. When they were placed underneath they looked away and fretted. We just put the gym aside and introduced it later.) When your baby starts to pull herself up, put the gym away, as it tips over very easily.

T I P   ➤ Make your own crib gym by suspending a solid bar or chain of plastic links across the baby's crib or playpen. Use plastic links to hang one or two colorful, noise-producing objects like measuring spoons, plastic keys, bangle bracelets, and rattles. Remove it when the playtime is over.

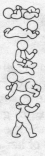

➤ There are also musical toys, such as the Dakin Paddy Whack musical clown, that hang from the playpen or crib side. You pull a ring and the baby is treated to a song. Later, the baby will be able to start the music herself. Some also make patterns of light on the ceiling.

➤ Activity mats combine a colorful, washable surface for the baby to lie on, with built-in toys—usually a mirror, some sort of dangling toy, a noisemaker, and something to chew on.

GENNY: *During Kara's first year, we always traveled with her activity quilt—especially if we were going to visit friends who didn't have little ones. Aside from ensuring a familiar, clean, padded place for Kara to play, if she threw up, it was on our quilt and not on their Oriental rug.*

► Bigger, bolder rattles. Now that your baby can grasp them by herself, transfer them from hand to mouth to hand, and shake them, she'll probably take to them with greater enthusiasm. Soft vinyl toys and teethers are ideal. The Tracking Tube (sold by *Parents* magazine) and rattles with fabric bodies and bright faces such as Wiggle Worm (also sold by *Parents*) are good choices. Look for a multicolored, multitextured, noise-making toy with an animal face.

► Roly-poly toys that tip over and pop right back up.

► Keys: stick to a plastic set of bright, clacking ones.

► Activity centers or busy boxes offer a variety of actions and reactions, from rudimentary to fairly sophisticated. For now, the baby will like to watch you perform the tasks. Soon you'll be able to guide her hand so she can do them herself. Once she can sit up, you can attach the toy to the side of her crib or playpen. The Fisher-Price Activity Center is a good choice. Ambi's Play Time busy box is small, portable, and can be carried around like an attaché case. Smaller busy boxes work well on strollers and car seats.

T I P ➤ You can prolong your baby's toys' appeal if you keep them fresh. Change the objects dangling from a mobile or put an outfit and a hat on Teddy. You can also rotate your child's toys to keep up her interest in them. That musical clown that was so exciting for the first three weeks and then became invisible will regain its appeal after a few weeks' vacation in the closet. In fact, there's no reason why three or more families couldn't purchase a quantity of toys as a group and rotate them every month or so.

TOYING WITH THE TELEPHONE

 The game is to make up phone conversations. Pretend to be talking to Grandpa or one of your baby's buddies. Have a chat with Old MacDonald or Raggedy Ann. Use your imagination and talk to the sun, a school bus, or a sea turtle. Some babies will delight in listening to others chat, and some babies will want to do the "talking" themselves. Listen to the way babies imitate adult voice patterns and telephone habits. It's amazing what little minah birds they are.

For safety's sake, most play telephones have really short cords, which can be frustrating for the baby because the whole telephone lifts up when she picks up the receiver. You can cut off the cord entirely and throw it away. As a rudimentary puzzle, periodically show your little operator how to reunite the telephone and receiver.

Of course, the one problem with toy telephones is that kids assume (and consume) all your phones, toy and authentic. If you want to keep your real telephone equipment working, you have to draw distinctions between your phone and hers. Your best shot is to

➤ Keep working phones out of reach.

➤ If yours is one of those babies who insist on having the real thing and you decide to give in, make sure the phone is disconnected and the cord is no more than six inches, or remove it altogether.

➤ Make the baby's phone "just for Baby" and the working phone "just for grownups." Good luck.

LAURIE: *Anna had four telephones before her first birthday—a plastic rotary dial model, a cordless with musical buttons, a one-piece unit, which was a great traveling companion and, yes, finally, a real one. Deciding to make do with one less extension proved a good move. She was in heaven and the battles over our phones ended.*

SIGHTS FOR WATCHFUL EYES

Until your baby is mobile—soon, very soon—you can give her some extra-special visual treats:

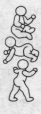

➤ Puppets: use a store-bought one or improvise with a sock or napkin. Draw little faces on your index fingers. Make the puppet talk or sing in any variety of pitches, or make it trip, fall, or smack into something, a baby's idea of high comedy.

➤ Inflatable barrels, with bells and balls inside, to roll on.

➤ Bubbles, the kind you blow through a wand, for the baby to watch and bat.

➤ Plastic shake-up snow domes.

Sitting Baby Toys

Once a baby can sit unassisted, the options for her playtime increase tremendously.

JIL: *When Jenny began sitting, we'd prop her up on the floor and surround her with fuzzy animals. She'd hold court, chatting with one, then another, delighted to be the center of their attention. Finally a use for all those stuffed toys!*

Now that her hands are free, your baby can actually start to use toys independently, although not for long periods. Many of the toys popular at this stage develop hand-eye coordination and manual dexterity.

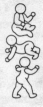

➤ Blocks are just right for sitting babies. There are the standard wooden ones as well as plastic, cardboard, rubber, and sponge (avoid the sponge variety with babies who can't resist chewing on them). There are fabric-covered foam blocks, squeaking blocks, alphabet and picture blocks, and stacking and nesting blocks. Her first blocks should be big enough for her to hold in two hands and may get smaller as she develops more dexterity (see Chapter 4, "Fun & Games" for ways to play with blocks). Fisher Price First Blocks are small, colorful plastic shapes and very versatile: they come in their own container, which has a top that is also a shape sorter. (Be sure you buy the set that has square, circular, and *triangular* openings in the top. The one with the square, circular, and *rectangular* openings is tough even for well-rested adults.)

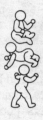

➤ A stacking toy, such as the one with the multicolored plastic doughnuts that fit over a spindle that we all had as kids, is a fine addition to your toy chest at this age. Fisher Price makes them with five rings or seven; the pole untwists from the base for easier storage or travel. The rings are lightweight; they spin, roll, and are great in the bath. They make nifty teethers, bracelets, anklets, and hats.

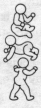

➤ Bead mazes come in all shapes and sizes. They're freestanding contraptions of colored beads that the baby moves along a twisting, turning roller coaster of coated heavyweight wire.

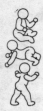

➤ Plastic nesting cups or boxes are good fun (see Chapter 4, "Fun and Games", for why). Some brands come with animals imprinted on the bases, which can be used for making sand prints, too. Gowi makes a neat set of large decorated cups that comes with a shape sorter.

➤ Most pounding benches require more arm strength than an under-one can manage. But Ambi's Hammer Bang! is a nice one that a sitting baby can work. The baby hits one of several multicolored balls, which then roll down a little chute and pop out the bottom.

T I P ➤ Put a toy in each hand of a sitting baby and then offer her a third. At around six to eight months, she'll soon catch on that she must put down one toy to get the third.

➤ Anna had a wooden peg toy in which four pegs fit into springed, color-coordinated holes. She *loved* this toy but also found the pegs were perfect "cigars" for her Groucho Marx impersonation. Make sure pegs pass the "choke" test. Play with peg toys must be monitored and the toy put away when not in use.

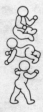

➤ Pop-up toys such as Playskool's Busy Poppin' Pals were a hands-down favorite with all our kids and held their interest way past their first birthdays. Animals or "Sesame Street" or Disney characters pop up from under little doors when the baby pushes a button, turns a knob, pulls a lever, or rotates a dial. At first, your baby may not be able to manipulate all the gadgets herself, but meanwhile she'll love seeing them pop up when you do it or guide her hand. (*Caveat emptor:* some models of this toy have sticky catches.) A good old jack-in-the-box will teach the same sort of cause-and-effect lesson; the traditional crank-operated ones are tougher for a baby to operate solo and scare many little tykes.

Crawling Baby Toys

Once your baby is mobile, her main entertainment will be seek-and-destroy missions. Toys take second chair to all the *objets* that so far she's been able to see but couldn't get her mitts on. When she's inclined, she'll still play with her sitting baby toys. When you want to engage her newfound mobility or other motor skills with something new, try:

➤ Balls (see Chapter 4, "Fun and Games," for types and specifics).

➤ Large wind-up toys, which are fun for her to chase and pounce on. Playskool's push-and-go cars and trucks, and animals that a baby can set in motion herself are especially entertaining.

➤ Farms and houses with animals or people that go in one door and come out another are a toy that your baby may start to play with now. They earned our award for inspiring the longest sustained periods of independent play (seven minutes, easy) and the pieces can be used in other ways as well (in her second year, Molly used the farm animals with her Duplo set). The Fisher Price Animal Sounds Barn is our first choice in farms (when the baby opens the doors, an unseen cow moos, which delighted Sam and made Annie belly laugh but terrified Jenny) and the Little Tikes Play House for homes.

➤ Wheeled vehicles with little people, animals, or moving parts are a thrill. Pushing them and crawling after them is a great game.

Toys for Cruisers and Walkers

Once your baby is on her feet (cruising with or without your help or walking on her own), there are some toys that will be especially captivating to her:

➤ Push toys, which are usually modeled after cars, fire engines, buses, wagons, and such, feature is U-shaped bar in the back on which the baby can steady herself while she goes through the motions of walking. Some come with buttons, levers, knobs, and other activities that turn them into oversize busy boxes. We liked the versatile ones that could also be ridden on. Be sure to check the height of the seat; if it's too short, your baby will soon outgrow it and may trip over her own feet. Another option is one with a storage compartment under the seat. This appeals to babies, and it is also a handy repository for grown-up essentials. (Look here first when you can't find your keys or glasses.)

HEDY: *I bought Molly a little train to ride or push that made an impossible-to-ignore choo choo whenever it moved. My pals thought I was crazy for having it in my apartment, but I could always tell how far away Molly was by the volume and how fast she was going by the tempo. When she was riding it and I hadn't heard a choo choo in a while, I knew it was time to investigate.*

➤ Pint-sized shopping carts are also push toys and fun for the baby to tote her "stuff" around in. The Playskool Steady Steps Walker Cart comes with a plastic juice bottle, jam jar, and milk carton and has a real advantage in that you can lock its wheels; some of these toys can go awfully fast and frighten brand-new toddlers.

➤ Babies push the classic Fisher Price Corn Popper as if it were a vacuum cleaner or pull it along behind them. Where the bag would be is a plastic see-through dome in which colorful beads pop when the toy is pushed. The clatter makes this many a child's favorite companion on walks.

➤ Musical instruments that amuse babies at this stage are toy pianos, maracas, drums, xylophones, tambourines, and hand bells. Bambina makes a line of brightly colored plastic instruments in animal shapes. A small battery-operated keyboard that you can buy in a discount audio appliance store makes a great first-birthday gift.

T I P ➤ If the baby figures out how to open the battery compartment of any toy, tape it securely closed. Never let a baby suck on a battery; the acid, should it leak, is toxic.

➤ Crayons: children have trouble staying in the lines. Babies have trouble staying on the page. They all have trouble keeping the crayons out of their mouths. However, when you think she can be taught not to gnaw on them or to draw on the one freshly painted wall in your home, it's time for crayons. For most families, that will be next year. Little hands can work the oversize ones most easily. Put a vinyl tablecloth down and weight or tape the paper so it stays in one place.

Toy Storage

Once a child has entered your life, your home is not likely to make it into _House Beautiful_ for a while. Some level of disarray is unavoidable. You'll inhibit your child's pleasure by hovering over her and straightening up after her as she moves from toy to toy. If play is your baby's job and toys her tools, think of your home as her workplace.

In the dark of night when the moon is full, toys multiply and divide. The rings fall off the pole and the animals spill out of the barn. Babies cannot "see" toys that are in a jumble—even though they delight in making the jumble. To begin with, take a few minutes every day to tidy the baby's toys. (Or assign this job to your spouse or caregiver.) Put the rings back on the pole and the little animals back in the barn. When your baby is old enough to start making her own selections, it's much easier for her to play when her toys have all their parts together.

Of course, your baby's toys will need to be in her view and in reach. And, you'll probably require some semblance of order in your life. Most of us chose to accomplish both these ends by turning the bottom shelf of the changing table, low shelves in wall units, and the bottom compartments of entertainment centers into toy storage.

We then organized the blocks and balls in see-through stackable bins, multicolored plastic mesh baskets and boxes, shoe boxes, the containers that wipes come in, and the like. Those of us who kept most of the baby's toys in the living room preferred cabinets with doors. That way, when the toys were "asleep" for the night, the living room didn't look like a toy store on inventory day.

A toy chest is another possibility. The advantages are that pickup is uncomplicated, the toys are out of sight, and it can be decorated with cute designs. The disadvantage is that the toys are all piled on top of each other, making them hard to get at and rendering it impossible to keep a toy's pieces together. If the chest has a lid, be sure it won't unexpectedly slam shut on baby fingers. Ventilation holes are essential.

LOIS: *We used a big cheap styrofoam cooler for Annie's toys in her first year. By the end of the year, it had been destroyed by Annie and her pals' efforts to get the toys out, graphically demonstrating to us how useless a toy chest is from a baby's point of view.*

Stuffed animals present a different sort of storage challenge. You'll likely have more of them than your baby could play with in her lifetime. Line them up on high shelves and think of them as a decorative element. Or buy either of two products marketed especially for this purpose: a toy hammock, which you hang in a corner, or a a plastic chain with attached clips, from which you suspend the critters (see the "Mail Order Sources" appendix for the last two).

When I Was Kid . . .

Toys are great fun. But a hangar full of state-of-the-art playthings is not essential. George's all-time favorite toy his first year was a plain old ball. Sam always carried a handful of toothbrushes when going out in his stroller. Molly preferred a ring of keys when she wanted to play. Children thrive as well with two or three safe, age-appropriate toys as with a dozen of the newest, most expensive inventions.

6

FOR A SONG

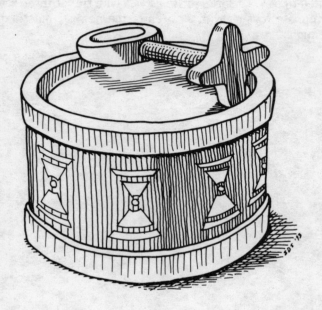

In utero, babies tune in to the timbre of their mothers' voices, reverberating heartbeats, and the rhythmic rocking their mothers' movements create. It's only natural that sound and rhythm—the basic components of music—are an intrinsic part of a newborn baby's world.

Parents all over the world coo, hum, and sing to their newborns to express their love. Long before we can use language to communicate with our children, we can reach out to them with music—even if we're not on our way to Carnegie Hall.

LIBBY: *There Sam was, a soft, warm baby lying in my lap on our first night home from the hospital. I was overtaken by the urge to sing to him but hesitant: my voice is B-A-D! The first tune that came into my head was "My Guy." Sam's milky blue eyes widened, but he didn't call for the usher to throw me out. I then hobbled through "You Are My Sunshine." Still no tears. I've sung him to sleep practically every night since.*

Oh Say, Why Sing?

Before he can respond to anything else, your baby will be captivated by the familiar sound of your voice. They love it all—humming, whistling, talking, or singing—this last, a loosely defined term that covers everything from sing-talking like Rex Harrison or M. C. Hammer to reciting Mother Goose with great expression, to raising your alto voice to a falsetto soprano that your baby seems to like.

You don't need a full repertoire of patented "baby songs." Anything will do: "Happy Birthday," a national anthem, an advertising jingle, your school or camp song. It's all music to your baby's ears. (Nonetheless, we have scattered lyrics to songs throughout this book and collected many of them in the "Words to Songs" appendix.) In fact, you don't even have to sing a "real" song. You can sing "I love you, I love you, even though you smeared cereal on my new shirt, I love you" at different tempos, in different voices, to different tunes. Just "hum a little hum," to quote Winnie the Pooh.

T I P ➤ Few of us can remember more than a couple of old favorites in their entirety. We know the first couple of lines, then trail off into a sort of mumbling-humming combination. Don't worry about it.

We found ourselves breaking into song at many different times for many different reasons. Use music to add some fun when you

➤ Want to play. New babies aren't yet ready for so many things. But they are receptive to facial expressions, and songs are particularly good at helping people loosen up and get goofy. It's nearly impossible to sing a song or recite a rhyme impassively.

➤ Want to teach him first words and sounds. Songs, with their repeated refrains and innumerable opportunities for naming people, places, animals, feelings, and worldly things are a perfect medium for learning what the horse says, how this old man comes rolling home, and how to say "I love you." At the end of the year, you'll be able to capitalize on each new word he learns by singing every song you can think of in which the word of the week is key.

➤ Need to alter a cranky baby's mood. There's an unwritten law that requires babies to become cranky just when you need them to be their most good-natured. Breaking into song just when your child's brow starts to furrow can help him forget, even if only for a few precious minutes, about the crying jag he was about to start.

➤ Are trying to establish routines. Nothing is more comforting to babies than routines. The more familiar an act, the less balky the baby. Songs, if incorporated into your daily routines ("This is the way we wash your hair" or "There's soup in your bowl, Dear Kara, Dear Kara") can be particularly useful in that they lend familiarity to an activity even when it occurs away from its usual place.

➤ Need to alleviate fear. Well-loved songs are helpful in any situation in which a baby's sense of security is threatened—being dropped off at day care or traveling to Grandma's, for example. This is because your voice conveys reassurance to the baby and the song itself is comforting in its familiarity.

➤ Want your baby to go to sleep. Ah, yes. Singing a baby to sleep is one of the most tender and cherished human traditions. Some lullabies have been handed down through so many generations that it's impossible to trace their roots. The themes are the same in every language: it's the quiet, dark time called night; I'm here and you are safe; sleep sweetly; we love you. There's a special joy in crooning the same songs to your baby that your parents, grandparents, and baby-sitters crooned to you.

T I P ➤ Some babies may perk up rather than nod off when they're sung to. For them, humming, droning, chanting, or even whistling a lullaby may prove more successful. George stuffed a fist in Paula's mouth whenever she started to sing him to sleep, preferring to fall asleep in silence.

No matter how much you like a song, singing it over and over and over and over can be really boring. You can certainly learn new songs, or you can improvise on what you already know. Add a new phrase or reference. Rewrite a rhyme. Incorporate the baby's name. See if the baby notices that you've switched to a new, perhaps completely incongruous word. For instance:

> Hush little baby
> Don't say a thing
> Daddy's gonna buy you
> A yo-yo string.
> And if that yo-yo string goes snap
> Daddy's going to buy you a folded map.

or

> I know a girl whose name is Molly.
> Marcus likes to call her Molly Polly.

There are other good reasons for becoming inventive and substituting your own lyrics in songs. Simply, you may find them objectionable, violent, sexist, or racist and want to get an early start on helping your child grow up free of such things. There were, each of us found, certain lyrics we couldn't bring ourselves to sing.

JIL: _I've always hated having the baby fall out of the tree at the end of "Rock-a-bye Baby," so instead I sing: ". . . when the bough breaks/the cradle will fall/and down will come baby/into Mommy's arms." I know it doesn't rhyme, but Jenny didn't seem to notice._

LAURIE and GENNY: _When we come to the end of "Baa Baa Black Sheep," half the time we sing, "One for the little boy who lives down the lane, the other half, "One for the little girl who lives down the lane." Same goes for "Ten Little Indians."_

HEDY: *In order to avoid singing about dying to Molly, I changed the ending to "There Was an Old Lady Who Swallowed a Fly" from "perhaps she'll die" to "perhaps she'll cry."*

LOIS: *In our house, the old woman who lived in a shoe with so many children she didn't know what to do, "kissed" them all soundly and put them to bed.*

ALWAYS A CRITIC

Babies like more than "children's" songs. Try classical music, rhythm and blues, swing, jazz, country, gospel, show tunes, reggae, rock and roll, big band tunes, or bebop. Leave your preconceptions about what makes good "baby music" behind. Introduce your baby to your favorite artists and see if your child is as captivated by them as you are. Be prepared, however. He may not tap his feet to any of the selections you choose. His taste may not be the same as yours, or he may not yet be a music lover.

LIBBY: *When Sam was seven weeks old, I left him, nervously, with a baby-sitter. I was sure I'd come home to find his eyes red from crying. To the contrary, Sam had sacked out soon after the sitter had turned on a tape of Gregorian chants she'd brought with her. "Babies like it," she explained.*

As he changes from one developmental stage to the next, your baby's taste in music may change, too. George preferred soothing love songs for his first two or three months, then wanted to jive with more rhythmic stuff (see the stage-by-stage listings later in this chapter).

T I P ➤ If you have the equipment (and the time—fat chance), make your own tape by recording parts of records, tapes, or discs once you zero in on the types of music your baby likes best. Jenny's dad made a rock and roll tape that she loved to "dance" to as soon as she could pull herself up.

STARTING A MUSIC LIBRARY

When choosing recorded music for your baby, remember that you're going to hear these songs more times than you can possibly imagine. Don't buy anything that makes you wince. Even the songs you thought were pretty snappy at first will wear on you as time goes on. Songs you disliked to begin with will make you crazy.

And don't limit your search for songs to records, tapes, and compact discs. Some of our favorite tunes are emitted by talking geese, teddy bears, music boxes, musical pillows, mobiles, wind-up crib and stroller toys, and tiny electronic keyboards. (If you plan to use the toy to help the baby go to sleep, make sure that the music plays for several minutes or more and that the winding mechanism isn't too loud.)

JIL: _It seemed as if Jenny's dad hated every new cassette I bought for Jenny. Finally I came upon Sharon, Lois & Bram, and lo and behold, we all liked them. I packed up most of the other tapes and, one by one, bought the complete works._

So that you don't end up with a discard pile the size of Jil's, take the following steps to familiarize yourself with baby music:

➤ Before purchasing a recording, try to borrow it (or another by the same performer) from a friend or the library.

➤ Consult reviews of children's recordings for clues to what's popular. Ask a librarian to help you find publications in which these appear. Even if a recording is highly touted, go for a test run before purchasing.

➤ If your baby can't get enough of a cassette, you may be inclined to run out and immediately buy the whole _oeuvre_ of the artist. Don't. Whatever it was that appealed to your baby at the moment he decided he liked the music may not hold up on subsequent purchases. Bring home one at a time.

➤ Try and keep a running list of what titles you already have so that you don't wind up with several tapes with all of the same songs on them.

HEDY: *When I wanted Molly to get used to falling asleep listening to a cassette instead of my singing her to sleep, I gathered up the many recorded versions of "Twinkle, Twinkle" (the only song she wanted me to sing to her at bedtime) we owned, intending to make a "Twinkle, Twinkle" tape just for her by alternating the different versions along with my own voice. I never got around to it, but I still like the idea.*

Once you're ready to shop, you may have some trouble; children's departments in large record stores usually offer slim pickings. We've been lucky with the following sources:

➤ bookstores (both children's and the larger chain stores)

➤ toy stores

➤ television—sometimes there are offers for a big collection of children's standards for not so big a price

➤ mail-order catalogues (see the "Mail Order Sources" appendix)

A handful of performers have a veritable monopoly on the children's music market. We've found it's hard to go wrong with:

➤ Raffi

➤ Sharon, Lois & Bram

➤ Fred Penner

➤ Tom Glazer

➤ The Children's Television Workshop, a.k.a. "Sesame Street"

➤ The many volumes of Disney Songtapes, treasure troves of old favorites

➤ The Best of Disney in four volumes

There are also some more unusual recordings that will both broaden your child's musical experience and give you a break from "Old MacDonald." Here are some names to look for (title first; then artist; then distributor or source):

➤ *All For Freedom*; Sweet Honey in the Rock; Music For Little

People (see the "Mail Order Sources" appendix). This renowned female a capella group breathes new life into popular standards and lesser-known traditional songs.

➤ *Peace Is the World Smiling*; various artists; Music For Little People (see the "Mail Order Sources" appendix). Well-known musicians (Taj Mahal, Pete Seeger) sing children's songs on this tape. Part of the proceeds from sales go to charity.

➤ *Growing Up Together* and *Pulling Together*; Gemini; 2000 Penncraft Court, Ann Arbor, MI 48103; (313) 665-0165. Sandor and Laszlo Slomovits, entertaining twin brothers, sing some old standards and original tunes.

➤ *Make-Believe Day*; Rory; Alcazar Productions, Inc. (see the "Mail Order Sources" appendix).

➤ *Disney's For Our Children* (to benefit the Pediatric AIDS Foundation); various artists; most record stores. This tape of old favorites was recorded by a remarkable lineup of artists (Paula Abdul, Bob Dylan, Little Richard, James Taylor, et al.).

➤ *American Folk Songs for Children*; Pete Seeger; Smithsonian/Folkways Records (distributed by Rounder Records, 1 Camp St., Cambridge, MA 02140; (617) 354-0700). One of several Pete Seeger recordings for children.

➤ *Disney's Sebastian*; the Caribbean crab from *The Little Mermaid* sings "Day-O," "Jamaica Farewell," and other island tunes.

➤ *Disney's Beauty and the Beast*; the sound track from the movie, which will enjoy plenty of adult airtime, too.

Music for the First Year

In the first year of his life, even the mundane seems new and interesting to your baby. Because music is abstract and a baby's ability to grasp anything abstract is one benchmark of his growth, music provides a particularly informative peek into your child's expanding intelligence.

A newborn just gazes at the source of the sounds. A lap baby will begin to anticipate the next phrase after you've sung the first notes. A sitting baby may make an effort to clap when he hears a favorite tune. A crawler is physically able to get a tape (if you're crazy enough to leave them in reach) and hand it to you when he's ready for an afternoon with the Pops. And as the year comes to a close, a cruiser will begin asking—in one way or another—for favorite themes and come to understand that "moo" is what the cow says, and not just a funny noise.

Newborns

 What songs should you start off with to make a pleasant impression on those tiny ears?

In his vulnerable first weeks, the sounds of the world can be an ongoing assault to your newborn's senses. You've probably noticed how often your baby startles at what seem to you like the most ordinary sounds. Soothing music like gentle lullabies or love songs can calm his skittish nerves. Blues and torch songs of the forties seem to have just the right lilt for some babies.

Grown-up Music for Kids

➤ "Old Paint" and "Blue Bayou"; Linda Ronstadt; *Simple Dreams*; Elektra/Asylum Records.

➤ "I've Got a Crush on You" and "Someone to Watch over Me"; Linda Ronstadt; *What's New*; Elektra/Asylum Records.

➤ "Little Cowboy"; Harry Nilsson; *Aerial Ballet*; RCA Victor/Dynagroove.

➤ "It Had to Be You," "Always," "What'll I Do," and "As Time Goes By"; Harry Nilsson; *A Little Touch of Schmilsson in the Night*; RCA Victor.

➤ "Pennies From Heaven" and "Let's Put Out the Lights and Go to Sleep"; *Pennies from Heaven*; Warner Brothers Records.

Some of our favorite recordings of lullabies for newborns are listed below. Addresses for hard-to-find items are included; the rest are usually available at music, book, and children's stores.

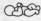

> *Earth Mother Lullabies from Around the World (Volumes 1 and 2)*; Pamela Ballingham; Earth Mother Productions, Inc., Box 43204, Tucson, AZ 85733; (602) 575-5114. Unique and beautiful lullabies are recorded in native languages from many countries.

> *Lullaby Magic*; Joanie Bartels; Discovery Music. Bartels's beautiful voice is recorded on one side; the other side features instrumentals-only versions of the same songs.

> *Sing with Me Lullabies*; Blane and DeRosa Productions; Random House. Soothing versions of tried-and-true standards.

> *Nitey-Nite*; Patti Dallas; Golden Glow Recordings. Another well-known collection of old favorites.

> *Heartsong*; Steven Bergman, Box 4577, Carmel Valley, CA 93921; (408) 624-4556. The very sweet melodies on this tape make soothing background music.

Old Favorites for Newborns

(See the "Words to Songs" appendix for some lyrics.)

> "Hush Little Baby" (The Mockingbird Song)

> "Amazing Grace"

> "Swing Low, Sweet Chariot"

> "Rock-a-bye Baby"

> "Taps"

> "Sleep, Baby, Sleep"

> "Kumbaya"

LAP BABIES

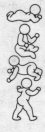

One of the real joys of this period is the first appearance of your child's sense of humor. At last, you've found your audience. You string a series of nonsense syllables together and make a funny face, and he smiles. Then you smile and laugh. Then he laughs. The sounds and sights that you notice tickling your baby's funny bone are insights into his unique personality. These early glimpses are truly wondrous. See Chapter 4, "Fun and Games," for chuckle-producing suggestions.

PAULA: *Both my kids loved an old camp song, "The Cannibal King" (see the "Words to Songs" appendix for lyrics). What the cannibal king does was completely lost on them, but when the king sings, "Ba-room, Ba-room, Ba-room, ba-dee-a-dee-yay," and when each ba and room was accompanied by a kiss on the belly, toes, or nose, it never failed to bring on peals of laughter.*

To help get your toes tapping and your knees bouncing, here are a few suggestions for songs to sing to your laughing lap baby:

Old Favorites for Lap Babies

(See the "Words to Songs" appendix for some lyrics.)

➤ "Row, Row, Row Your Boat"

➤ "Twinkle, Twinkle, Little Star"

➤ "Rain, Rain, Go Away"

➤ "Ten in the Bed"

➤ "You Are My Sunshine"

➤ "The Grand Old Duke of York"

➤ "London Bridge"

➤ *Morning Magic*; Joanie Bartels; Discovery Music. This is a tape of contemporary and traditional wake-up songs.

➤ *Animal Songs and Sounds*; Fisher Price. Nursery rhymes, animal sounds, and songs like "Pop Goes the Weasel" made this Molly's favorite.

SITTING BABIES

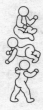

Although they still seem so, well, babyish, sitting babies understand a lot of what is going on around them. During this stage, your baby will not only delight in the songs you sing but will actually come to recognize the most familiar ones, given only the first few bars. With much waving of his arms and legs, he'll eagerly anticipate the melody that follows.

You'll continue to sing many of the songs you've already been singing to him, but you will notice a distinct difference in his response. Though you'll still have to clap his hands for him or hold his arms over his head when the sun comes out to dry up all the rain, your baby clearly understands that the movements go with the song. In fact, some babies at this age even try to make the motions themselves and can succeed with a little help from you.

LOIS: *When Annie was nearly two, we bought a cassette that included the song "Hush, Little Baby." When the song came on, she crawled into my lap, sobbing, "I want my mommy." I was stymied. My confusion only grew when she asked me to replay it several more times, sobbing less and less and managing to explain: "I don't want Daddy to hold me. I want Mommy sleepy-peepy" (her word for going to sleep). "Not Daddy." She saw that I still didn't understand and was clearly frustrated. Then her face lit up. "Nummy!" she said (her word for nursing). Now I was even more at a loss. She hadn't nummied in quite some time. "Nummy. Sleepy-peepy. I want my mommy," she repeated.*

Suddenly I remembered: When Annie was six months old, I'd decided to stop bringing her into bed and nursing her when she awakened during the night. I remember listening as Annie's dad walked her back to sleep in the next room, quietly crooning, "Hush, Little Baby." It couldn't be. I asked her, "Do you remember this song?" She nodded. "Daddy carry Annie. But I want Mommy. I want to nummy." By then, however, her sadness had taken a backseat to the excitement she felt about being able to make herself understood.

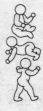 This is also a good age to try a live performance on your little music lover. Go to a park or mall and find someone strumming on the ol' banjo or playing any other instrument. In many cities, you stand a good chance of coming across musicians in subway and train stations, in parks and plazas, and on busy street corners. Or take him to an outdoor concert or a rehearsal for a concert; just position yourself so you can make a quick exit if need be.

By now, your baby will begin to give you clear indications of which songs he prefers. When you sing a tune on his top-ten list, he'll wriggle from head to toe; songs that don't strike his fancy will be met stony-faced.

LAURIE: *Once she could talk, Anna shouted, "No" whenever anyone dared to sing one of her nonfavorites, and kept it up until they knocked it off. But she'd listen to her favorites over and over. At Anna's insistence, her grandfather sang "Georgie Porgie" so many times that she started calling him Georgie . . . and still does.*

Though you won't want to abandon the songs you sang before, you can augment your repertoire with

➤ "Hey Dum," "A, You're Adorable," "Peanut Butter," "Three Little Monkeys," and "Chirri Bim"; Sharon, Lois & Bram; *Smorgasbord*; Elephant Records.

➤ "Marvelous Toy"; Peter, Paul and Mary; *Peter, Paul and Mommy*; Warner Bros./Seven Arts Records.

➤ "What Does Baby Hear?" "What Does Baby See?" "Bye Bye" and "Baby's Bath"; Tom Glazer; *Music For Ones and Twos*; CMS Records.

Old Favorites for Sitting Babies

(See the "Words to Songs" appendix for some lyrics.)

➤ "Bingo"

➤ "He's Got the Whole World in His Hands"

➤ "Eensy Weensy Spider"

➤ "I'm a Little Teapot"

➤ "Baa, Baa, Black Sheep"

➤ "Pop Goes the Weasel"

CRAWLING BABIES

 It's as if a light bulb clicked on in his head. All of a sudden, he's trying to make the gestures you've been showing him for the last nine months or so. At times—can it be?—it seems as if he's trying to sing along. Now you're becoming a team. This is truly one of the high points of parenthood and, given your baby's enthusiastic response, of babyhood, too.

Your baby's leaps of understanding during this stage will increase his enjoyment of songs about animals and the sounds they make, the parts of his body and the movements they make, and the everyday tasks they accompany. Even the routines your baby frets about seem to go a little more smoothly when you make a song in which your baby can participate. Once he's able to stand on his own two feet, he'll practically be asking you for the next dance.

JIL: _I always sang, "Now we'll put the toys away, the toys away, the toys away" when we cleaned up at the end of the day. Mind you, Jenny paid no attention to this whatsoever, nor did I expect her to. I was hoping for a subliminal effect, and I think I got it. When she was two, Jenny started helping me pick up when she heard me sing the tune._

PAULA: *George also knows this song. However, when I break out my rendition, he takes out the toys I put away. I'm taking lessons from Jil.*

Here are some additions to diversify your crawling baby's collection:

➤ "Baby Beluga"; Raffi; *Baby Beluga*; Troubadour Records, Ltd.

➤ "Wheels on the Bus" and "Going to the Zoo"; Sharon, Lois & Bram; *Elephant Show Record*; Elephant Records.

➤ "Abba Dabba Honeymoon" and "Dance to Your Daddy"; Sharon, Lois & Bram; *Singing 'n' Swinging*; Elephant Records.

➤ "These Are Baby's Fingers"; Bob McGrath; *The Baby Record*; Golden Music.

Old Favorites for Crawlers

(See the "Words to Songs" appendix for some lyrics.)

➤ "This Old Man"

➤ "Animal Fair"

➤ "Where Is Thumbkin?"

➤ "Old MacDonald"

➤ "Skinnamarink"

➤ "Teddy Bear's Picnic"

CRUISING BABIES

 By the time your baby is cruising, he is on the threshold of a burst of verbal development. Many of his first words will, in fact, be learned through songs. He'll ask for a favorite with a word or gesture that he never uses for anything else.

At first you may not understand your baby's unevenly phrased requests. He may stubbornly repeat his message until you get it. If you don't understand that "rounarounarouna" means he wants you to sing "The Wheels on the Bus," he may think to add the paddle wheel hand gesture that accompanies the "round and round" part to help you out.

LOIS: *When Annie was eight months old, I took her to see our next-door neighbor, a cellist. He gave her a private concert of a beautiful piece of classical music. Annie adored it and waved her arms and legs throughout. After that, she'd "sing" an approximation of the first notes whenever she wanted to go knock on Steve's door.*

At that moment when you finally understand what he's asking for, both of you will shriek with delight and you'll no doubt sing the song with unusual gusto. Even a song you've sung too many times sounds new and exciting the first time you sing it on request.

HEDY: *Just before Molly's first birthday, she seemed fascinated by songs with lots and lots of verses. She loved for me to sing "The Green Grass Grew All Around," "Would You Like to Swing on a Star" and "Little White Duck." I didn't mind a bit because I love them, too.*

New tunes to introduce at this point include:

➤ "Fuzzy and Blue" and "All By Myself"; *Surprise! The Sesame Street Muppets*; Sesame Street/Children's Television Workshop.

➤ "Everybody Wash," "Rubber Duckie," "La-La-La," and "W"; *Bert and Ernie Side by Side*; Sesame Street/Children's Television Workshop.

➤ "Sesame Street"; *Sesame Street I* Original Cast Recording Sesame Street/ Children's Television Workshop.

➤ "Artichokes" and "Mommy's Girl"; *Marcia Berman Sings Malvina Reynolds' Rabbits Dance*; Marcia Berman B/B Records.

➤ "The Cat Came Back"; Fred Penner, *The Cat Came Back*; A&M Records/Shoreline.

➤ "Peter and the Wolf," Serge Prokofiev; various recordings.

Old Favorites for Cruisers

(See the "Words to Songs" appendix for some lyrics.)

➤ "The Alphabet Song"

➤ "There Was an Old Lady Who Swallowed a Fly"

➤ "Head, Shoulders, Knees, and Toes"

➤ "If You're Happy and You Know It"

➤ "The Hokey Pokey"

➤ "Over in the Meadow"

I Want My MTV

Music videos. Hmmm. This is a gray area. In their first year, most babies aren't ready to appreciate videos, although there are always exceptions. If the baby pays attention to the musical portions of "Sesame Street," he may be ready for the video age.

To gauge your baby's interest, borrow a children's music video from a friend with an older child or the library and see how your baby reacts. If the program holds his interest for more than a second or two, it's time to buy or rent your own. Start with a video of your baby's favorite songs performed by a real live musician so your baby will be able to see the instruments being used to make music. If there are babies in the audience, so much the better. Buy a few and borrow a lot is a good rule of thumb for videos at this stage.

As with recordings, whenever you can, preview videos before buying. Rent a new one now and then from your local video store or review the collection in your local library. Trading videos with other parents is another good way to preview, and this will expand your video library without shrinking your wallet. Don't trade a tape that your baby seems really attached to, though. It'll make for rough going if he somehow manages to indicate that he wants it and you can't produce it. Wait till he's seen it a hundred times and his interest wanes.

T I P ➤ Tape episodes of "Sesame Street," "The Elephant Show" (Sharon, Lois & Bram's program), "Lambchop's Play-Along," and so on. Kids _like_ watching these over and over and over.

When you're ready to buy, you'll discover that children's videos are not nearly as difficult to find as musical recordings. Children represent a big portion of the video market, so you're likely to find them at

➤ video stores (look for gently used tapes at video rental shops)

➤ large drugstores

➤ five-and-dimes

➤ supermarkets

➤ department stores

➤ toy stores

➤ bookstores

➤ mail order catalogues (see the "Mail Order Sources" appendix)

Here are some of our favorites:

➤ _Raffi in Concert; A Young Children's Concert with Raffi; Raffi;_ A&M Video/Shoreline.

➤ _Disney's Sing Along Songs;_ Walt Disney Home Video; a several-volume collection of songs and the scenes in which they were sung taken from the Disney films.

➤ _Sing Yourself Silly;_ Sesame Songs/ Children's Television Workshop, Random House Video.

➤ _Rock & Roll;_ Sesame Songs/ Children's Television Workshop, Random House Video.

➤ _Baby Songs;_ High Tops Video; lots of footage of babies doing baby stuff.

➤ _Kidsongs;_ View-Master Video; there are several volumes including one called "A Visit to Old MacDonald's Farm" with lots of animals in it.

➤ Anything from Sharon, Lois & Bram.

➤ *Gymboree*; Warner Home Video.

Some parents look down their noses at others who introduce videos to their children at this age. Other parents see videos as a cultural bonanza for their babies. Since videos haven't yet been proven critical for, or detrimental to, development, make your own choice.

PAULA: *By the time George was cruising, a Raffi video would keep him occupied long enough for me to boil spaghetti for dinner. Children's music videos didn't exist when my first child was born; life sure was easier the second time around.*

Don't be afraid to try your baby on music videos. For now, the sounds are what captivate him; next year the sights will grab him as well. The point is that it's music to his ears; his happy responses are music to yours.

7

BOOK 'EM

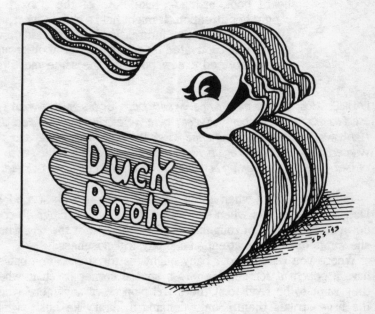

In her first few months, books won't be any fun for your baby except perhaps indirectly—as a source *you* might refer to for the words to a nursery rhyme. In the next few months, pictures of all sorts will start to fascinate her. Then, sometime in the second half of the year, she'll make a connection between words and pictures. That's when books are ready to join her other toys.

Books will help your baby absorb the words for what she sees, how she feels, and what she wants, in itself a form of play. We all noticed, for example, that some of our babies' earliest words were drawn from the books they liked to hear. For you, books will become an ideal way to give your baby the undivided attention she adores—and the few stationary moments you crave.

Ready to Read

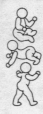 Forcing a child to look at books before she is interested in them is counterproductive, so don't bother. You'll know that your baby's ready to "read" when her hand passes by a rattle and picks up a board book instead. Take note of the book that caught her attention. It might hold a clue to what will fascinate her in the future. Each of our kids, we noted, was captivated by one subject or another and always greeted a new book on the same old topic happily.

LAURIE: _Most of the time Anna would push books away when we tried to read to her in her first year. There were only two she liked, Jan Pienkowski's_ Shapes _and Katherine Ross's_ The Little Noisy Book, _and she wanted these again and again. My guess is she didn't like the passivity of being read to, preferring activities in which she could participate._

Take note also of when in her day she stops to look at a book. Does she like books when she wakes up in the morning? To cool down after a round of roughhousing? At the end of the day when she wants one-on-one attention and physical closeness?

Where you read to your baby might matter, too. Some babies have a penchant for settling into a special corner or chair when they want to be read to. Others will plop down anywhere when the urge strikes them. Some demand a librarylike hush, while others can abandon themselves to a book regardless of the mayhem around them. Pick up on her cues.

You can then use reading in other ways—to entice her away from another activity, as a distraction, to calm her down, to help her get ready for sleep, or to make her sit quietly when you are tired.

HEDY: _When it came time for me to teach Molly to fall asleep without nursing, books (and songs) were key. Instead of snuggling against me for milk, she'd snuggle in for a couple of stories with a bottle instead._

Your baby will find other uses for books as well. She'll chew on them (Jil used to tell people that Jenny "devours" books), talk to them, stack them, and sit on them. She'll explore the physicality of books and use them as steps, ramps, tunnels, building blocks, and UFOs.

Your baby may insist that her favorite book be toted from crib to car seat to stroller, much as another child won't go anywhere without her special blanket or bear. For her, the book is a source of emotional comfort.

T I P ➤ If your baby has a hand's-down favorite, buy another copy and hide it away. Sooner or later the original will get lost, drenched, or come unglued. If you never use the extra, you can always give it to another child as a gift.

Since she is learning by repetition, she'll want to read the same book over and over again—long after its appeal has worn off for you. Try a new book on the same topic, from the same series, or by the same illustrator.

LIBBY: *I never thought anything positive would come from my having memorized Sam's books by reading them over and over and over. But once, stuck on a stalled, dark train, I amused him by reciting his favorites to him. Sam thinks it's funny that I can read to him without his books, and it's gotten us through many a traffic jam and grocery store line.*

How to Build Up a Library

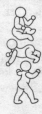 The number and variety of children's books is daunting, no matter how book oriented you are. Until you become familiar with the most popular titles, characters, authors, and illustrators, the shelves before you will seem forbiddingly crowded. Especially for the beginning of the first year, stick with books that

➤ have large, bright illustrations

➤ depict familiar subjects

➤ have no more than one or two words on a page

➤ have words in easy-to-read type (for learning the alphabet next year)

➤ are made of cardboard or heavy stock (the pages are both more durable and easier for small fingers to turn)

➤ don't cost more than a few dollars

Later in the year you can get a little more sophisticated and start reading books with real story lines.

T I P ➤ Sometimes on the copyright page of a book, buried in the text where all the copyright and other publishing information is clustered, there is a one-line summary of the book. Some books also note the appropriate age. Ask the sales clerk or librarian for help.

Discovering where your baby's taste in books lies requires her participation. Watch her as she plays with other children's books, and see which ones attract her. When you go visiting, talk with parents and sitters about the books that have gone over big in their households. (Book choices are also a great conversational ice-breaker.)

Experiment with types of illustrations and different artistic styles. Some babies show a marked preference for photos; others prefer drawings. Most will be attracted to simple line drawings in primary colors. More subtle drawings become interesting after age one.

You may acquire a starter library from gifts, hand-me-downs, and those treasured volumes that survived your childhood. Before adding to these with a vengeance, take some time to get to know what you've got, what's available, and—most importantly—what you think will tickle your baby's fancy.

Thumbs Up

How do you know which books are best? If you're unsure, awards are useful indicators. Look for a seal or notation that the book has won one of these four major annual book awards:

➤ Randolph Caldecott Medal (for illustration only)

➤ Boston Globe-Horn Book Awards (two for text, one for illustration)

➤ The New York Times Choice of Best Illustrated Children's Books of the Year

➤ John Newbery Award (one award for text and illustration combined)

Many other book awards are given annually by magazines, parenting organizations, and library associations. Reviews of children's books also appear in children's and parenting magazines and in Sunday newspaper book sections. Awards and reviews, however, shouldn't determine your choices. At this point, go with what you and your baby like.

LIBRARY TIME

 You can get a broad view of the range of titles by visiting the children's room of your local library. Dare you attempt a visit to that haven of quiet and risk being chased out in a windstorm of ssshes? Sure! Children are always welcome in the children's rooms. Other reasons to go:

➤ There's a librarian to help you figure out where to start looking.

➤ Your baby will be able to "shop" for new titles, and you can look at as many books as you like for as long as you like without buying them. Just make sure the baby doesn't teethe on them.

➤ You'll meet other parents who can share titles of their children's most coveted books; in fact, some libraries allocate certain hours for parents and babies.

➤ You can acquaint yourself with the library programs that will be available to your toddler the next year.

➤ If you've already made your picks, you can test your selections on your child before making commitments at the bookstore.

➤ Some have toys and simple puzzles for babies whose literary yearnings have not yet blossomed.

WHERE TO SHOP FOR BOOKS

For those who are lucky enough to have one nearby, a children's bookstore offers the widest selection and the most knowledgeable help. The books are usually arranged conveniently with "first books for babies" shelved together.

When you're choosing, don't judge a book only by its cover. Read the entire book before purchasing it. The first two pages may enchant, but the last two may offend or be scarier than you think appropriate. For example, Babar's mother is killed by a hunter. Peter Rabbit's dad is turned into rabbit pie. You decide.

Other book sources are

➤ general-interest bookstores

➤ department stores

➤ toy stores

➤ five-and-dimes

➤ museum shops

➤ children's gift shops

➤ supermarkets

➤ newsstands

➤ stationery stores

➤ catalogues (see the "Mail Order Sources" appendix)

➤ thrift shops, yard sales, library book sales, etc.

Children's Book Clubs

Some of us thought these were great—and still think so—because the store comes to you with a select group of new (sometimes discounted) books to choose from regularly. Here are the names of some popular ones:

➤ Britannica Home Library Service, Inc., Box 6268, Chicago, IL 60680-9961; (800) 323-1229.

➤ Children's Book-of-the-Month Club, Camp Hill, PA 17012; (800) 233-1066.

➤ Books of My Very Own (a division of Book-of-the-Month Club, Inc.), Camp Hill, PA 17011-9849; (800) 233-1066.

➤ Dr. Seuss Book Club, Grolier Enterprises (Attention Premium Department), Sherman Turnpike, Danbury, CT 06816; (203) 796-2560.

➤ Sesame Street Book Club, Golden Press, 120 Brighton Road, Clifton, NJ 07015; (800) 537-1517.

JIL: *I recommend waiting until your child is a little older to join a book club so she can be excited about getting a package. Also, if you join too early, you're going to have a huge library before she's three. Finally, it's often hard in those early months to get it together to return the monthly selection if you don't want it.*

LIBBY: *Instead of bringing back ordinary souvenirs when I visited Australia, where my parents are from, I brought back classic children's books and placed them in my mother's care. Now, when we visit Granny, Sam and his little sister, Eliza, are treated to stories about jackaroos and wombats read in her authentic Aussie accent. Keep an eye out (and ask others to do the same) for interesting editions when you travel.*

Baby's books don't have to be expensive. If you're looking in an aisle where all the volumes cost upward of $10, ask the clerk where the "other" baby books are. Many of our babies' favorites cost between $2 and $5. (Golden Books are still a bargain at under $2 each.)

T I P ➤ Check local bookstores and libraries for information on book sales, mailing lists, readings, and special events for kids.

SELF-MADE BOOKS

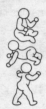

You don't always have to buy books in order to build your library. Making them yourself is another option.

PAULA: *Will still pulls out his tattered copy of* Mommy's Away, *which I made for him before leaving for two weeks when he was eighteen months old. Because it was made of construction paper and hand-stitched,* Mommy's Away *was always read with adult supervision. It's now preserved in an envelope along with Will's birth certificate and newborn footprints. I just regret not making it out of sturdier paper.*

It pays to think about materials before putting a lot of effort into making a book because, if it survives, it will someday become a family heirloom, treasured by your child long after other books have been forgotten. Meanwhile, she'll treat it as roughly as any other book.

You can use fabric, wood, cardboard, or paper for the pages. Create your own pictures or cut them out of magazines, books beyond salvage, or bad books with good pictures. Family photographs make great illustrations; babies are fascinated by pictures of themselves and familiar faces. Our kids each have their own small-format albums of their friends, relatives, pets, and selves at various stages. Paula found a key ring with room for photos at a dimestore, and now George won't part with it.

JIL: *My sister-in-law lives in California, while the rest of her family is on the East Coast. She wanted her son to be able to recognize his relatives when they visited, so she made a family book by sealing each picture in a plastic bag, which she'd flip through with her son before and after family reunions.*

Right now the baby is too little for complicated story lines. Stick with subjects she's familiar with (Fido's Day) or that she'll want to remember (Kara's First Trip to the Zoo). Be as simple or as elaborate as you like, and don't worry about professional results. No matter what you do, the book will be very dear to you and your baby.

You can find something that your baby will like to look at in almost any publication. In fact, she may take a shine to other sorts of printed material long before she'll sit on your lap and look at a book.

LOIS: *One day, just after Annie learned to crawl, I came back from the kitchen into the living room, where I'd left her, and found that she was gone. After a moment of panic, I looked for her in her room. Not there. More panic. I looked in my bedroom. There she was, absorbed by a page of minuscule text in one of her dad's veterinary journals.*

Other sources of "reading matter" are:

➤ mail order catalogues of children's products (Annie preferred Hanna Andersson and After the Stork)

➤ the pictures on food packaging (Molly had a fondness for the Green Giant)

➤ calendars

➤ greeting cards

➤ playing cards

➤ magazine advertisements

➤ maps

➤ the comics

GIVE ME BOOKS, LOTS OF BOOKS

 When asked what you need for your new baby, and you already have enough receiving blankets to swaddle Dumbo, encourage this generous soul to buy books. You may receive a handsome edition of

Alice in Wonderland or *The Adventures of Tom Sawyer*—lovely though not immediately practical gifts. In case you're asked for specific suggestions, here are some types of books that are right on the mark:

➤ vinyl foldout books

➤ board books

➤ pop-up, peekaboo, and other activity books

➤ song books

➤ books that turn into mobiles (bookmobiles!)

If you'd like to ask for particular authors or illustrators, here's a list of the ones we liked best for our babies' first year:

- Don Freeman (the Corduroy series)
- Eric Hill (the Spot series)
- Dick Bruna
- Norman Bridwell (the Clifford series)
- Jan Pienkowski
- Richard Scarry
- Margaret Wise Brown
- Helen Oxenbury
- Eric Carle
- Phoebe Dunn
- Tana Hoban

KEEPING THE BOOKS

Building your baby's library is only half of the task; keeping the books from being loved to death is the other. This is one of those situations in which the best defense is a good offense. Here are a few suggestions:

➤ Check out the book's structural integrity before you buy it. You needn't pretend you're in a Samsonite luggage commercial, but check the spine and pages to see if it's sturdy.

➤ Run a piece of tape vertically (up and down) between the pages at the spine.

➤ Put a piece of tape where pop-up parts meet the page, and avoid designs that pull off or break easily (giraffes' necks, for example).

➤ If you want to preserve the illustrated paper covers, it's best to remove them. (You can hang them in the baby's room, if you like.) They rip easily and won't survive your baby's hands-on reading efforts.

T I P ➤ If you remove a book's dust jacket and are left with a bare cover, use stickers that relate to the story to make the book more recognizable to you and your baby.

Try as you might, you can't reinforce feathers that stick up out of duck heads, bits of fabric that lift up for peekaboo games, and other fragile decorative elements. If they don't get eaten or lost, you can try to put them back on with glue, double-sided tape, or, in the case of bindings, needle and thread (many librarians are trained resewers and are happy to teach others the craft).

No matter how skillful your repairs, sooner or later there will be fewer feathers and peeks that will never boo again. Seeing the serious wounds of their books disturbs some babies. When a book gets to the point of no repair, it's time to bring out the reserve copy or make a special trip to the bookstore together for a new one. Don't throw the old one out in your baby's presence.

Books for the First Year

 Developmentally speaking, your baby will become a new person every few months; the books you choose should advance along with her, too. Nonetheless, keep the old ones around. As she grows and rereads them, she'll discover new meanings in their pictures and words. And they're wonderful for those sentimental journeys.

How do you know when she's ready to move from faces to simple pictures or from words to a simple story line? Try one of the newer sort. Tell her a little story (the drama of the little teapot is plenty). What did she think? You'll know.

T I P ➤ If you find yourself with a baby bibliophile, keep mini-libraries in various rooms around the house, especially by telephones. And keep a brand-new book or two hidden away to use as a fun distraction when your baby is at the end of her rope.

Similarly, use your judgment when deciding how many of these selections you plan to buy. If you've got a book lover, you might want all of them and then some. You may find that a small handful of new ones at each stage is plenty.

Columnist Anna Quindlen wrote a lovely article about how thrilled she was when her children began taking real pleasure in reading entire books on their own. She ended the piece by saying that she only hopes that her kids will grow up to live in homes where there are never enough shelves to store their books. We all heartily agree.

NEWBORNS

  Your newborn might be quite receptive to certain printed images, especially high-contrast graphics (the line where dark meets light is what gets them). In truth, black-and-white vinyl foldouts (see Chapter 5, "Toy with Me") are probably the only best-sellers on a newborn's reading list.

Keep the short-term nature of this developmental phase in mind when shopping. You can borrow, use your arts-and-crafts skills (stick a couple of crossword puzzles to pieces of cardboard), or hang up your old checkerboard instead.

Nursery rhymes are ideal for newborns. Like babies, they're short and sweet. Although you won't sit down to read an entire volume of nursery rhymes with your baby for a while, keep the tome handy. Newborns are soothed by the repetitive rhythm of rhymes. Like songs and games, nursery rhymes are diversions you'll pull out of your hat whenever you need a momentary entertainment throughout your baby's early years.

Our favorite nursery rhyme anthologies include:

➤ _The Little Dog Laughed and Other Nursery Rhymes_ by Lucy Cousins (New York: E. P. Dutton, 1990); includes 53 rhymes illustrated in color in a childlike style.

➤ _A Treasury of Mother Goose_ by Hilda Offen (New York: Simon & Schuster, 1987); includes 163 rhymes, some illustrated in color.

➤ _Mother Goose, the Classic Volland Edition_ by Frederick Richardson (New York: Rand McNally, 1971); with almost 300 rhymes, this one is the most exhaustive collection to be found.

➤ _Richard Scarry's Best Mother Goose Ever_ by Richard Scarry (Racine, Wisc.: Western Publishing Co., 1970); each of the 50 rhymes is illustrated in Richard Scarry's signature whimsical style.

➤ _The Orchard Book of Nursery Rhymes_, chosen by Zena Sutherland, illustrated by Faith Jaques, (New York: Orchard Press, 1990); includes 77 gorgeously illustrated rhymes.

➤ _The Baby's Bedtime Book_ by Kay Chorao, (New York: E. P. Dutton, 1984); an exquisitely illustrated collection of 27 traditional nursery rhymes, poems, and lullabies share the common theme and are arranged to mimic increasing sleepiness.

LAP BABIES

Once your baby has moved on from her fairly limited newborn routine, she'll complain for a new reason—she's in need of stimulation. This is the time to move on to her first true books.

Babies in this stage are most fascinated by the human face and the myriad of emotions it expresses, which is why making funny faces is usually good for a laugh. There are two books that are simply accordion-style foldouts of faces. The _Let's Look Book_ (see Chapter 5, "Toy with Me") is one. The other is _Mrs. Mustard's Baby Faces_, which is made of laminated cardboard and features happy baby faces on one side and unhappy baby faces on the other.

Animal faces are great, and especially fun for babies when you accompany the pictures with the corresponding sound effects. When you get tired of the same old moo, baa, and quack, look for books or wildlife magazines featuring more exotic species.

Books that incorporate different textures and sounds (some have noisemakers sealed within the pages) go over big with lap babies. At first you'll need to guide the baby's fingers over the pages, but soon she'll be able to press, pull, and push them herself. *Pat the Bunny* is a classic example of this type of book. First published in 1942, it has simple activities young babies like. It's available with a toy bunny, too.

HEDY: *Somehow* Pat the Bunny *never made it into my childhood; I thought it was about a bunny named Pat. A similar one, the* Touch Me Book *was one of my earliest favorites. I loved watching Molly discover the bumpy, scratchy, sticky textures for herself, just as I had more than twenty years before.*

In addition, your baby might like to listen to any book in which the text is pleasantly lyrical, even if the words are way beyond her and the pictures less vivid than most favorites. There's a board book series of Beatrix Potter's *Tales of Peter Rabbit* that many babies—and parents—love.

We have put together lists of books our kids enjoyed and arranged them developmentally. However, our experiences introducing different titles at different stages varied tremendously. Our suggestions are meant to give you some direction; use your instincts when making selections.

BOOK LIST FOR LAP BABIES

➤ *Mrs. Mustard's Baby Faces* by Jane Wattenberg (San Francisco: Chronicle Books, 1989).

➤ *Pat the Bunny* by Dorothy Kunhardt (Racine, Wisc.: A Golden Book/Western Publishing Co., 1942).

➤ *The Touch Me Book* by Pat and Eve Witte (Racine, Wisc.: A Golden Book/Western Publishing Co., 1961).

➤ *Soft as a Kitten*, illustrated by Audean Johnson (New York: A Random House Touch-Me Book, 1982); a touchy-feely text like *Pat*.

books, vinyl books, and simple puzzles; there is a stuffed Spot, too; the farm animals in this book will be more appealing at this stage than the numbers.

➤ *Baby's First Counting Book* (New York: Platt & Munk/Grosset & Dunlap, 1988); it's not the numbers that make babies like this one; it's the large animal picture on each page.

➤ *Baby's Words*, photographs selected by Debby Slier (New York: Hello Baby Book/Checkerboard Press/Macmillan, 1988); good shots of basic objects babies encounter daily.

➤ *Ernie's Bath Book*, illustrated by Michael J. Smollin, (New York: Children's Television Workshop, 1982; vinyl); a nice way to get babies into a bathtub frame of mind with Sesame Street's wise-cracking character.

➤ *Mommy and Me* by Neil Ricklen (New York: A Super Chubby Book, Little Simon, Simon & Schuster, Inc., 1988; also in the series: *Daddy and Me, Grandpa and Me,* and *Baby's Friends*); bright, colorful photos of really cheerful adults playing with really cheerful babies.

➤ *Zoo Animals* (New York: Chubby Board Books, Little Simon, Simon & Schuster, 1982; one in a lengthy series); cartoonlike drawings of exotic animals.

CRAWLING BABIES

 Your crawler's on the move now, interested in exploring her environment—opening doors, peeking in boxes, and finding out what goes on in the corners of the house she hasn't been able to visit before. The books she is drawn to will reflect this. All of a sudden, she'll love to read about eating, bathing, crawling, and clapping—the very activities she's mastering.

LOIS: *One evening, soon after Annie started crawling, her dad tried to play a joke on her. "Annie, go get* Anna Bear's First Winter," *he said to her as he elbowed me and winked. She went straight to her pile of books, shoved them around, and crawled back victorious. We never*

again assumed that she was looking at the pictures individually rather than taking in the whole book.

To make her explorations even more exciting, hide favorite books in unexpected places; put her chunky ABC on her walker tray or on the seat of her stroller. It's also time to find some novelty books with snaps, wheels, pop-ups, and other moveable parts that give her something to do as she looks at the pictures. And consider sitting down together with a book when your crawler has crawled as much as she possibly can for one day but can't stand to quit.

LAURIE: *Anna loved* Big Bird's Big Book. *It's about three feet tall and two feet wide (four feet when opened flat). Each page is a delightful tangle of Sesame Street characters engaged in related activities. She'd search the pages for each character and, placed upright or in an A-frame, it doubled as a playhouse for her.*

This is the time to try out books about animals so the baby can see the picture of the animal, hear its name, and the sound it makes all at the same time. Books about body parts are good choices, too.

BOOK LIST FOR CRAWLING BABIES

➤ *Big Bird's Big Book*, illustrated by Joe Mathiew (New York: Random House/Children's Television Workshop, 1987).

➤ *Look, Baby! Listen, Baby! Do, Baby!* by True Kelley (New York: E. P Dutton, 1987); really funny drawings of babies involved in all sorts of activities.

➤ *I Can* by Helen Oxenbury (New York: Random House, 1986; also *I See, I Hear, I Touch*); the same round-faced children as in the aforementioned Oxenbury series, but now they're on the move.

➤ *Baby's First Words*, photographs by Lars Wik (New York: Random House Chunky Books, 1985); photographs chronicle a sweet , androgynous baby's day.

➤ *The Very Hungry Caterpillar* by Eric Carle (New York: Philomel Books, 1987; also, *The Very Busy Spider* and *The Very Quiet Cricket*); there's also a palm-sized version of this modern classic about a caterpillar's metamorphosis into a butterfly.

➤ *Good Morning, Little Bert*, illustrated by Norman Gorbaty (New York: Random House/Children's Television Workshop, 1987); Bert wakes up, gets dressed, eats breakfast, and plays.

➤ *Who Sees You on the Farm* by Carla Dijs (New York: Grosset & Dunlap, 1987; also set at the zoo, at the ocean, in the forest); these are pop-ups, so they can take only so much wear and tear, but the colors are vivid and the pop-ups really do pop up.

➤ *Big Red Barn* by Margaret Wise Brown, illustrated by Felicia Bond (New York: Harper & Row, 1989); by the same author as *Goodnight Moon*, this one follows a barnyard full of animals through their day.

➤ *Moo, Moo, Peekaboo* by Jane Dyer (New York: Random House, 1986); farm animals peek through cutouts while you read rhyming text.

➤ *Clifford's Animal Sounds* by Norman Bridwell (New York: Cartwheel Books, Scholastic, Inc., 1991 [one of a series]); the simple antics of a little red puppy (based on *Clifford the Big Red Dog*) for older readers.

➤ *Here Are My Hands* by Bill Martin, Jr., and John Archambault, illustrated by Ted Rand (New York: Henry Holt, 1987); a nicely illustrated rhyming introduction to the parts of the body.

➤ *Baby's First Body Book* by Maida Silverman, illustrated by Robin Kramer (New York: A Little Poke and Look Book, Grosset & Dunlap, 1987; also *Baby's First Finger Rhymes* and more); sweet cartoon toddlers show how they use the different parts of their bodies.

CRUISING BABIES

 If you were struck by your crawling baby's independence, you'll be tempted to hand over the car keys to your cruiser. She may prefer—or insist on—picking out the books you read to her and may even drag one over to you when the urge to read strikes her. She'll certainly demand to turn the pages herself or to have you do it in exactly the right way. Even if she's not on her own two feet yet, the connections that she began making a few months ago between words and the world become more and more plentiful every day.

If your newborn had (and liked) a face book of family photos, she'll appreciate it in a whole new way now. Watch her study it and wait for the spark of recognition that lights up her face when she realizes, "I know who that is."

During this stage, books that follow the progression of day to night within the text can be especially handy. These sorts of stories make wonderful prenap and nighttime reading because they mimic the child's encroaching drowsiness and set the mood for sleep, something that cruisers may resist.

T I P ➤ Before-bed or nap stories are best read in your high school science teacher's monotone. Save the enthusiasm for other times of day.

Displaying another developmental leap that often occurs at the end of the first year, your baby may try to parrot the words that are most meaningful to her from a well-loved book. As speech becomes a new focus, animal and noise books will rejoin object and activity books on her top-ten list.

PAULA: *From nine months on, George had a thing for alphabet books. Nothing else pleased him. Forget about baby see or baby do. I thought the power of twenty-six letters would lose their allure but they never did. When he was two and a half, he was telling me that D is for devil and Z is for zebra. I've been instructed to keep my M for mouth shut.*

A visit to the doctor, being separated from a parent for a few days, angry feelings, a new pet, going on a trip—all of these potentially heavy situations can be softened by reading about them (several hundred times) beforehand or hearing a story you've invented.

Cruisers can be very hard on books and indestructibility becomes a priority now. Sturdy board books were made for this stage because they are used as roadways, tunnels, hats, missiles, steps, chairs, trays, and whatever else your creative little munchkin can think of. However, don't pull away her favorite volumes just because they're made of paper. A book that dies from an overdose of affection has died a noble death.

BOOK LIST FOR CRUISERS

 ➤ _I Can, Can You?_ by Peggy Parish, photographs by Marilyn Hafner (New York: Greenwillow Books/ William Morrow & Co., Inc., 1980); your baby can do the activities along with children in the book.

➤ _See What I Can Do_ by Patricia Linehan, illustrated by Laura Rader (New York: Grosset & Dunlap, 1990); a little girl and boy show off their agility to a rhyming text.

➤ _What Do Toddlers Do?_ (New York: Random House, 1985); a book of few words with great photographs of toddlers on the go.

➤ _Go, Dog, Go!_ by P. D. Eastman (New York: Beginner Books, Random House, 1961); antics of an army of dogs introduce basic words including colors, opposites, and actions.

➤ _One Fish, Two Fish, Red Fish, Blue Fish_ by Dr. Seuss (New York: Beginner Books, Random House, 1960; also _Mr. Brown Can Moo, Can You?_ and many more); classic Seuss rhymes and funny creatures for the youngest readers.

➤ _The Runaway Bunny_ by Margaret Wise Brown, illustrated by Clement Hurd (New York: Harper & Row, 1972); by the author of _Goodnight Moon_, this sweet story handles the whole moving away– touching base issue with kid gloves.

➤ *Tom & Pippo Take a Walk* by Helen Oxenbury (New York: Macmillan, 1989; also *Tom & Pippo in the Garden, Tom & Pippo's Day, Tom & Pippo and the Dog,* and more); with their engaging illustrations and simple story lines about familiar activities, these are perfect first story books.

➤ *Corduroy's Day* by Don Freeman, illustrated by Lisa McCue (New York: Viking Kestrel/Viking Penguin, Inc., 1985; also *Corduroy Goes to the Doctor, Corduroy's Party, Corduroy's Busy Street*); all feature Freeman's lovable bear, who's first learning about the world—just like your baby.

➤ *Wheels on the Bus* by Paul O. Zelinsky (New York: E. P. Dutton, 1990); the lavish illustrations in the book version of this musical standard make the song come to life. It even has wheels that go round and round.

➤ *Nursery Rhyme Peek-a-Book* by Eric Hill (Los Angeles: Price, Stern, Sloan Publishers, Inc., 1982; also *Animals, Opposites, Who Does What?*); the pictures in this series of books are brightly colored and the activities are fun.

➤ *The Peek-a-Boo ABC* by Demi (New York: Random House, 1982); especially small flaps sized for tiny fingers lift up to reveal a nickel in a nut, a queen under a quilt, and so on.

➤ *The Guinea Pig ABC* by Kate Duke (New York: E. P. Dutton, 1983); disarming, charming guinea pigs take advantage of the alphabet in new ways.

➤ *Anno's Alphabet* by Mitsumasa Anno (New York: Harper Trophy/Harper & Row, 1988); letters drawn as if made of wood with hidden surprises for the baby to find.

We were all "book people" before our babies were born. But now we're even more so, having realized that books are the perfect toys. They're cheap, they're safe, they're portable, they're versatile. They're great for amusing more than one child at a time, and they're well, fun.

8

ON THE ROAD

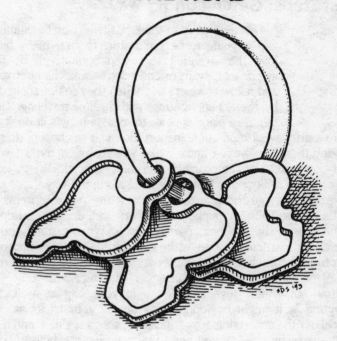

Travel? With a less-than-one-year-old baby? Sound impossible? It did to each of us, too. But for one reason or another, each of us found ourselves on the road, in the air, or on a train (and around the bend) with our baby at some point in that first year. A few of us traveled solo with our babies, some *en famille*. And you know what? We actually had some great times. Traveling with kids opens your eyes to new sights and experiences.

Given the diversity of grown-up and baby personalities and the ever-changing nature of your child's development in the first year, we can't give you a prescription for how to have fun on a family holiday. Instead, we're going to give you some general pointers about inventing fun while you travel (see Chapter 3, "Out and

About"), describe our favorite traveling games, recommend some toys that travel well, and direct you to some sources for information and advice.

First Steps: Getting Under Way

 Our first tip is to think positive. Don't assume the trip is going to be a disaster. In fact, many babies love the attention showered upon them by flight attendants, waiters and waitresses, chambermaids, and fellow travelers . . . when they're not zonked out by the action, motion, and thrill of traveling. Going to a new place appeals to many a baby's curiosity.

No matter what mode of transportation you've chosen, start by packing those things you know make your baby happy: a favorite rattle, animal, blanket, pacifier, teether, snacks. Bring extras because you're bound to lose something along the way.

Next, rummage through the toy chest for versatile items like nesting cups, balls, or puppets that work well indoors, outdoors, in the tub, in the sandbox, on the beach. When visiting another household, particularly one without children, you can improvise toys from the kitchen (see Chapter 2, "Domestic Bliss") and make use of "invisible" toys (see Chapter 3, "Out and About").

Stow some new toys and books in your bag as well. But, tempting as it might be, don't bring out all your tricks at once. Parcel out the entertainments—including songs, games, and magic tricks—one by one, as you need them, saving a couple of trump cards for the trip home. You may rely on most of your surprises during that interminable waiting-for-takeoff period and need none while in the air. If you find you've used all the new toys you'd stashed away just getting to Grandma's, buy some fresh ones for the way home.

T I P ➤ If you find yourself with some free time in an unfamiliar city, seek out a toy store or hands-on children's museum that permits babies to play with the toy displays. It'll be a pleasant change for your baby to spend some time with playthings other than the ones you've brought from home.

TEN LITTLE TRAVELING TOYS

 Between us, we've traveled to all kinds of places with all kinds of stuff. The best amusements to bring along are

➤ you (your lap, voice, fingers, etc.)

➤ a mirror

➤ peekaboo

➤ a squeaky, teethable toy

➤ an activity box

➤ puppets (which can include a face drawn on your hand with makeup or a pen)

➤ music (your voice, a radio, a personal stereo, piped-in tunes)

➤ snacks

➤ books, especially those with pop-ups or other activities

➤ nesting cups

PICKING A BABY-FRIENDLY VACATION SPOT

 The travel industry has caught on that folks with kids want hassle-free, one-stop, minimal-effort vacations. A good travel agent will be able to tell you about all-inclusive holiday options designed for family fun.

The answers to the following questions will indicate whether a particular hotel or resort goes out of its way to make a family vacation with small children as entertaining as possible:

➤ Are families welcome?

➤ Are the walkways paved? (Ever try pushing a stroller over sand or gravel?)

➤ Is there a baby-sitting or day-care service?

➤ Is there a baby pool, swing, or sandbox? If not, are babies welcome in the adult pool?

➤ Is there a playroom, a lobby, a fountain, a carpeted game room, or other public space where you can go with a baby for diversion? Even an ice machine counts (you can let the baby scoop ice and bring some back to play with in the bathroom sink).

Sources for Information

If you subscribe to parenting or travel magazines, keep an eye out for monthly columns and annual roundups of the best places to vacation with kids. In addition, Carousel Press publishes a catalogue of family travel books. Send $1 or a self-addressed, stamped envelope (with two first-class stamps) to Carousel Press, Box 6061, Albany, CA 94706. Or try one of the following books:

➤ *Great Vacations with Your Kids* by Dorothy Jordon and Marjorie Adoff Cohen (New York: E. P. Dutton, 1990).

➤ *Fielding's Traveler's Medical Companion* by Paula M. Siegel (our own Paula M. Siegel) and Eden Graber (New York: Fielding Travel Books, 1990).

➤ *The Candy Apple, New York with Kids* by Bubbles Fisher (New York: Prentice-Hall, 1989). And look for other destination-specific guides for kids.

➤ *Traveling with Children and Enjoying It* by Arlene Kay Butler (Chester, Conn.: Globe Pequot Press, 1991).

➤ *How to Take Great Trips with Your Kids* by Sanford Portnoy and Joan Flynn Portnoy (Cambridge, Mass.: Harvard Common Press, 1983).

Travel with Your Children (80 Eighth Avenue, New York, NY 10011; (212) 206-0688), a resource information center for parents and travel agents, publishes *Family Travel Times,* a newsletter on fares, packages, and dozens of other relevant subjects, ten times a year. Subscribers are also entitled to call Tuesday and Thursday mornings for over-the-phone advice.

LIBBY: *We went away when Sam was six and a half months old to what was advertised as a "family" vacation place. When we arrived, I found that all the activities and equipment were for older kids. I would have given anything for a bucket swing or a sandbox. Ask for specifics when you call for reservations.*

LAURIE: *On a trip to Tucson, we stayed with friends whose kids were already in school. One day, we brought Anna to their nursery school for show and tell. She loved the stimulation and attention.*

Car Trips

Although most young ones enjoy car rides, don't push your luck. The maximum amount of time an awake baby can be expected to spend in a car seat is an hour. Two is stretching it. You can

➤ Hang toys within reach of the baby (see Chapter 2, "Domestic Bliss"), or use an activity center that hangs from the back of the front seat (see the "Mail Order Sources" appendix); make sure the noises won't drive the driver around the bend.

➤ Play music (bring a portable tape player along if the car's not equipped with a radio or tape deck).

➤ Sing songs.

➤ Tell stories.

➤ Bring an older child (the entertainment committee) along.

If you're traveling with another adult, take turns driving so that you can alternate amusing the baby with clapping, body, finger and toe games, (see Chapter 4, "Fun and Games," and the "Words to Songs" appendix), and snacks in the backseat. If you're traveling alone, obviously, your ability to entertain the baby will be more limited. If you have no choice but to be on the road for hours and hours, try to plan the trip around the baby's normal sleeping rhythms, leaving at bedtime, for instance.

LIBBY: *Coming home from a long weekend away when he was ten months old, Sam was understandably getting cranky in his car seat. We'd sung every song, told every tale, and played with every puppet. It was too dark to see what was zipping by. Then we spotted the moon. It dodged the dark shadows of hills, trees, and clouds, tailing us the whole way home. Sam was rapt.*

Break up long trips with frequent rest stops, every 60–90 minutes (also for the benefit of the adult in the backseat). Keep an eye out for rest stops with playgrounds or fast-food restaurants with indoor play areas. Changing bambino's diaper while you slug back a cup of coffee won't do it. While you're out of the car:

➤ Give lap babies a chance to lie flat and kick.

➤ Give sitting babies some time on a quilt with a toy.

➤ Give crawlers and cruisers a chance to stretch their legs.

➤ Make body contact by cuddling, roughhousing, or sitting the baby on your lap while looking at a book or two.

➤ Buy a new toy at the gift shop.

Plane Travel

Plane trips, like other forms of motion, will often put your little one to sleep. If not, don't despair. When you consider airline travel from a baby's point of view, there's all manner of fun. You can

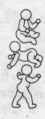

➤ Watch the planes taking off and landing from the observation deck while you wait to board.

➤ Talk about what's happening and mimic the noises of takeoff and landing.

➤ Count backward slowly as the plane begins its taxi down the runway and speed up as the plane speeds up, ending with an enthusiastic "Blast off!"

➤ Pay a visit to the galley.

➤ Break out the baby's favorite snack; pack a new one for him to try.

➤ Find the water fountain and give the baby a drink from one of those tiny cups.

➤ Go for a walk up to the pilot's cabin before takeoff.

➤ Find the other babies on the plane.

➤ Hold the baby's hand under the air-conditioning vent and turn the air flow on and off.

➤ Lift the ashtray lid or window shade a million times (don't do this with the meal tray; it'll drive the person in front of you nuts).

➤ Count "one, two, three" and fasten the seat belt so the baby can hear the click.

➤ Raise the armrests up and push them back down, letting the baby help.

➤ Look through the freebie in-flight magazine and make up stories about the pictures (this man is very unhappy because he has no hair; now he's very happy, yay!).

➤ Look out the window and talk about what you see.

➤ Visit the lavatory and wash hands, make faces in the mirror, apply lip balm, brush off crumbs, unwrap the tiny soap. Okay, now give the baby a turn. (Obviously, if the bathroom isn't clean, don't dally.)

➤ Engage the person behind you, if he or she is willing, in a game of peekaboo over the back of the seat. (Don't tell your nice neighbor that the game lasts an hour.)

➤ Give him little toys (they needn't be new) you've wrapped in tissue paper and ribbon to open.

HEDY: *When Molly was nine months old, we took a trip to Florida and our departure was delayed several hours. We'd walked—meaning I walked while Molly held my index fingers and toddled along—all over the airport and still had time to kill. Then we found a security checkpoint for carryon luggage that wasn't in use and spent half an hour or more rolling a small ball I had in my bag up and down the ramp. The moral: With a little inventiveness, you can manufacture a game anywhere.*

T I P ➤ Many books make two recommendations with which we take issue. 1) Reserving bulkhead seats does give you some extra room to maneuver, but there's no seat in front of you under which to stash your bag of tricks, and the armrests don't lift up. If the flight is relatively empty, you might be able to get an entire nonbulkhead row, complete with armrests that raise, to yourselves. 2) Preboarding allows you to get as much storage room as you need near your seat, but it also means a longer time confined on the plane.

Train Travel

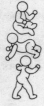 Many of the games we recommend for car or plane travel work well while riding the rails. The big bonus of train travel is that neither you nor your baby needs be confined to your seat. For parents of babies who hate to sit still, trains are a blessing. Some tips for rail travel:

➤ Inquire whether you can take a Superliner or other souped-up train to your destination. Some feature observation decks and multitiered sightseeing lounges. Some have music, movies, and cartoons.

➤ Try to snag seats that face each other for the added leg room, play space (bring a quilt along to put on the floor), and privacy.

➤ Choose seats near another family. Older kids generally love babies and will amuse your little traveler better than any toy.

➤ Look out the window for barns, animals, other trains, bridges, and other points of interest that will fascinate your baby.

➤ Let the baby push the button that makes the door between cars open (as long as neighboring passengers can stand the noise).

Grand Hotel Games

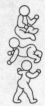 If your trip includes a stay in a hotel, here are some creative ways to capitalize on the amenities with your baby:

➤ Borrow a luggage cart, prop up the baby with bags, pillows, or blankets, and go on tour.

➤ Ride the elevators and escalators.

➤ Take a tour of the hotel, singling out what you don't see at home: crystal chandeliers, sparkling fountains, gleaming banisters, towering potted palms.

➤ Find an infrequently used carpeted staircase and let the baby crawl up and down to his heart's content.

➤ Visit the concierge, newsstand clerk, barber, or hairdresser.

➤ "Read" the brochures about local attractions.

➤ Hold the baby steady on a stool in the bar or coffee shop and spin, spin, spin.

➤ Explore the ballroom or convention spaces (when not in use).

➤ Show the baby how to collect some gravel from one potted plant and place it in the next. "Water" plants by placing an ice cube in each pot.

➤ Watch guests frolic in the pool or during an exercise class.

➤ Tinker with the newspaper, candy, and soda machines. Knobs, buttons, and little doors that move when the baby touches them are just new activity boxes.

The moral to our travel tale is: Do it! Don't stay home because you're afraid traveling with a baby won't work. It can, it will, and you'll be happy you went. *Bon voyage.*

9

PEER PLEASURE

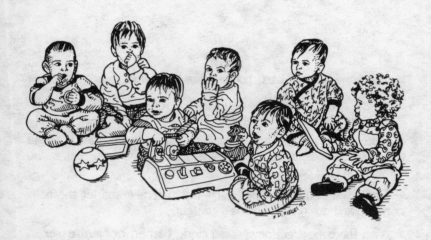

There are whole textbooks devoted to animals' primal need for company and companionship, and lots of parenting books that extol the benefits of socializing during the first year of a baby's life. We recommend it because spending time regularly with other parents of babies about the same age as yours will help you get through that challenging, thrilling, gratifying, draining, sometimes disorienting, scary period known as new parenthood.

Other parents (especially those whose babies are slightly older):

➤ understand exactly how you feel and will be supportive and reassuring.

➤ have mulled over all the same sorts of decisions you're consumed by and will freely share practical information.

➤ won't tire of your main subject of interest: raising baby.

➤ will usually be happy to hold the baby for a minute while you go to the bathroom all by yourself. Yahoo!

LIBBY: _I look forward to visiting friends with kids because I always learn something new: there's a book or toy I've never seen, a funny song I've never heard, a parenting technique I can try._

And besides, getting to a play date, class, or play group meeting gives you an incentive to get dressed and out of the house.

Babies Need Other Babies, Too

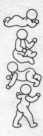

You aren't the only one who needs to socialize. In the course of her life with you, your baby will certainly become familiar with other adults. But what about getting to know other children? Play dates provide your baby with new experiences, new stimuli, and new faces. It's thrilling to see your baby come to recognize her friends and socialize with them. Through their early friendships, children begin to learn about common bonds, differences, tolerance, sharing, and love.

In her first months, your baby probably won't much care where she is. Once she's out of infancy, however, she will certainly revel in the good times she'll encounter at another baby's house. We believe that babies as young as six months start actively checking out kids their own age. Although she will notice and watch them, she won't "play" with the other babies, preferring parallel play. This is when two babies play side by side but without interacting with one another. No, it's not the same as a game of mah-jongg or water polo, but parallel play is play nonetheless.

FINDING NEW FRIENDS

 Where there's life, there are babies. And they have parents. Here are some ponds in which to cast your lines and reel in new friends:

➤ your obstetrician or pediatrician's waiting room

➤ the about-to-be-parents you met in your birthing class

➤ the parents you met where you gave birth, if you thought to exchange phone numbers (some clinics, birthing centers, and hospitals sponsor new parent get-togethers)

➤ shops and stoops in your neighborhood

➤ playgrounds, parks, libraries, and any other recreational facilities

➤ malls and supermarkets

➤ baby-equipment and toy stores

➤ places of worship

➤ parenting classes and lectures, including Red Cross classes

Don't hold back. If you're out and about and recognize that dazed new parent look and there's a baby nearby, you are looking at a potential new friend. Strike up a conversation. No need to be shy. Make a date to have lunch. Chances are the other parent will welcome your overture.

T I P ➤ Make a pen and notebook part of your basic stroller or diaper bag arsenal. Many contacts have been lost for want of something to write with.

THE FIRST DATE

 During your first year, when making any date involving another baby, bear in mind that

➤ It's not always so easy to get out of the door. Agree on a general time range as a meeting time.

➤ Nap time has different meanings for different parents and babies. Some babies are unpredictable and will fall asleep just before your scheduled play date. Some parents would want to keep the date anyway, while others would be thrilled to have the down time at home. Be honest about your needs and preferences to avoid misunderstandings.

➤ Meeting places should be easy, casual, and convenient. Starting out in someone's home often works best. (Note that if you have a pet, you should tell your guest beforehand. Similarly, if you're concerned about your host's having one, ask.)

➤ Parenting styles differ. Because the first year of parenthood is often full of insecurity and self-doubt, being with someone who does something in a way that you perceive as "better" or "worse" can be unnerving. Try not to judge your new friend, or yourself, too quickly or too harshly. You may still enjoy one another's company—and learn something from one another—even if your philosophies diverge.

➤ Ordinary Emily Post courtesy rules still apply.

MAKING EVERYONE—INCLUDING YOU—FEEL AT HOME

 When you're inviting people with children into your home regularly, whether singly or in a play group, it's a good idea to establish some ground rules and let them be known from the beginning. Obviously, you should strike a balance between your needs and those of your guests. The time you spend together will be more relaxing if the host isn't worrying about grape juice on the rug and the guests aren't wondering if a baby's teething on the remote is truly okay. Consider:

➤ Where are diapers to be changed? Do you mind if visitors dip into your supplies?

➤ Can visiting babies use your baby's high chair and/or crib? (Jenny has always been very possessive of her high chair, so no visiting child ever sits in it.)

➤ Is a baby (or an adult) with a runny nose still welcome?

➤ Where is food allowed and what kind of foods are acceptable?

➤ Is there any place in your house that's off-limits?

➤ Do you expect help picking up toys afterward?

➤ Is it okay if the visiting baby stands on your couch with her shoes on?

➤ What messy games (like bubbles) are allowed indoors?

➤ How will discipline be handled? (We recommend that parents talk to one another rather than scolding others' children themselves.)

OUTDOOR PLAY DATES

When a beautiful day beckons or the thought of spending one more minute inside is too much to bear, go farther afield to meet up with a friend. (See Chapter 2, "Domestic Bliss," for a list of possible destinations.)

A big advantage to meeting outside is that the host won't be tempted to straighten up before the guests arrive or be left with spills and piles of toys when they leave. The disadvantage is that outings can be more demanding in terms of planning effort and energy (rare commodities) on the part of the adults, and ultimately may not work out because of the weather.

T I P ➤ If a play date, whether one-on-one or with a group, is making you tense, something is wrong. Maybe your expectations aren't being fulfilled or the others aren't the right match for you. Make a change. Play dates are supposed to be fun.

Pay as You Play: Commercial Options

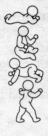 Play groups and classes organized by others are a great way for most babies to socialize. The options range from informal groups at local religious institutions, community centers, and universities to commercial national franchises. YMCAs usually offer an array of programs for babies. The quality, goals, methods, and degree of organization vary widely among programs—as do cost and class size. If a commercial operation interests you, arrange to attend a sample class or open house (which might be terribly crowded) with your baby before signing up. Bear in mind that the instructor you meet might not be the one who leads the class for which you sign up.

Some of the benefits of established play groups and classes compared with arranging play dates yourself are:

➤ They do the work of linking you up with other parents and caregivers of babies your baby's age.

➤ They aren't contingent on weather, last-minute changes in schedule, or a particular child's health.

➤ Having a specific place to go at a specific time adds some structure to your week.

➤ The instructors often know songs and games that you've never even heard of, and their enthusiasm is contagious.

➤ Some have toys and equipment your baby would not otherwise get to play with.

➤ They provide a safe yet challenging environment in which mobile babies can practice their budding physical and social skills.

When you discover that most of the activities in these classes go over equally well on the floor at home, you may question the investment ($3–$20 per hour or more). But will you actually mark off an hour a week to do nothing but play with your baby? Even if you do, you and your baby won't get the social benefits of a class or the laughs from watching a bunch of babies tumble around on a parachute.

To find out about classes, check the listings or advertisements in parenting publications (look for them in pediatricians' waiting rooms and baby equipment stores). Scan bulletin boards at supermarkets, toy stores, and children's bookstores. Or drop by local nursery schools and day-care centers for suggestions from staff members and parents. Local phone directories often have listings under the heading "gymnastics instruction."

T I P ➤ If you're thinking about a commercial play group only because you want to expand your repertoire of baby games and songs, there are video tapes available to inspire and guide you.

Classes are usually organized by the type of activity they stress, such as movement and physical play, music and rhythm, and swimming (music, in one form or another, is usually an element of all three types of program). Some organizations schedule combination classes so you can engage in two or more activities in one trip. Typically, classes last 45 minutes to an hour.

Gym classes are generally divided into

➤ A circle time during which everyone sits in a circle and sings songs, the first usually being an around-the-room hello song as a way of introducing the babies by name. Songs are usually accompanied by hand motions and other movements and increase in intricacy as the babies develop. It's basically a warmup period and gives the adults a chance to get to know each others' faces and the babies' names.

➤ A playtime during which the instructor guides the adults and babies as they use the equipment. Some instructors take an active role and organize one group game after another; some take more of a laissez-faire approach and encourage free play. (If your baby shies away from an enthusiastic instructor or is bored by one with a low-key style, consider switching to a class with a different instructor or dropping out for a while.) Expect a few minutes of one-on-one contact betweeen the instructor and your baby at each class.

➤ A cooling-down period during which you form a circle again, sing another song or two, and conclude with some form of good-bye song during which the babies are again addressed by name.

The two main commercial gym classes are

➤ Gymboree, a franchised play group with locations in many states (800) 222-7758. There's also a chain of Gymboree retail stores at which you can find out about classes in your area.

➤ Playorena, which has locations in New York, New Jersey, Connecticut, Massachussetts, Pennsylvania, and Florida (800) 756-PLAY.

Music classes typically include games with instruments such as bells and tambourines. The instructor may play the guitar or piano, sing unaccompanied, or use prerecorded music.

Swim classes at this age are usually designed to help babies feel at ease in the water within the safety of an adult's arms, not to teach them to dog paddle on their own. Instructors should be certified and there should be lifeguards on duty.

Remember the final sequence in _Three Men and a Baby_? Yes, there are actually classes where tiny babies are encouraged to swim in and under water. The proponents of this system believe that babies instinctively know how to swim and will do so when lowered or submerged in the pool. However, the American Academy of Pediatrics does not recommend this technique and neither do we.

Your baby's personality is the most important consideration to keep in mind as you decide whether to enroll in a class. If she thrives on bustle, she's likely to have a good time. If she loves to be tossed around, a gym class might be just the thing. If she's shy and startles easily, maybe she's not ready for a class yet but would love the company of other babies at a low-key play group in someone's home.

Assuming that you've decided that you want to enroll in a class, keep these factors in mind:

➤ Some _instructors_ have a background in early childhood development, which doesn't necessarily make them better than those who simply have a knack with children. Good ones make eye contact with you and your baby, are enthusiastic without being phony or forced, and have a flexible agenda. If you don't feel comfortable with the instructor, don't enroll.

➤ If *class size* is more than ten kids, the class can get a little out of hand; if there are fewer than four, you won't get a "class experience."

➤ If the *age range* is more than six months, it will be hard for the instructor to gear activities toward the class as a whole, given the fast-changing nature of development in the first year.

➤ *Class lengths* range from thirty to ninety minutes. If you have to travel a long way to get to the class or if your child takes a long time to adjust to new environments, a longer class may be the choice. If she's committed to her morning nap, a one-and-a-half-hour class may be too long for her.

JIL: *Just as Jenny was feeling comfortable in the forty-five-minute class I took her to when she was nine months old, it would be over. I adapted by arriving early and sitting on the sidelines of the earlier class so that by the time Jenny's class began, she was ready to participate.*

➤ *Cost* matters. Having to scrimp to afford the class will get in the way of your fun. Remember that these classes are not at all necessary for proper development. In fact, although most commercial programs claim that they are designed to enhance your baby's development, "designed to" doesn't mean "guaranteed to."

➤ Your *convenience* is important. If it's difficult to get to the location, you'll wind up skipping or resenting classes.

T I P ➤ Play groups and classes are meant to be fun. If you don't feel like going one day or sense that your baby doesn't, skip it, even though that feeling of "getting your money's worth" may be hard to ignore. Think zen. Let it go.

There are also classes that function as both entertainment for the babies and support for mothers. Mommy and Me classes, for example, organized by a local agency or individual, are divided into a play segment for the babies and a discussion segment, during which mothers talk and listen to each other, helped along by a trained counselor or social worker. During the discussion segment, the babies are supervised while they play by a second teacher or by one or two of the mothers, who take turns. Check the phone book to see if there's a group in your area.

LAURIE: *The "discussion facilitator" at Anna's Mommy and Me class was knowledgeable and down-to-earth. Talking to her and the other mothers was especially worthwhile because of the continuity of having the same group meet once a week. A side benefit was being able to observe and discuss our kids at play.*

The La Leche League, a national organization committed to encouraging mothers to breast-feed and supporting those who do, sponsors local group meetings. Technically, the meetings are a forum in which nursing mothers can discuss their breast-feeding-related concerns. Naturally all sorts of other parenting issues come up as well, and attendees share the benefits of any organized group of new mothers. Call (800) LA LECHE to find out whether there's a group in your area.

Forming Your Own Play Group

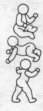 That's what we did. Libby and Hedy were the hub from which our group grew like the spokes of a wheel. They'd decided to form a play group, having tested out and been unsatisfied with several existing neighborhood options. We'll trace the path that led to the formation of our group so you'll get the general idea.

Libby lived in the same building with Hedy; Sam was born in January; Eliza was born three years later.
Hedy lived in the same building with Libby; Molly was born in March.

Lois happened to chat with Libby at the local bus stop; Annie was born in January.

Laurie knew Lois since forever and met Hedy and Jil at a local mom and tot group; Anna was born in March.

Genny once lived next door to Libby; Kara was born in August.

Jil shared a dorm room with Hedy; Jenny was born in April.

Paula met Hedy at the local greengrocer; George was born in January; her older son, Will, was six.

After a couple of false starts, we all wound up at Hedy's one October Friday afternoon, and it turned out to be a nice way to kick off the weekend. The crawlers crawled and the others lay on quilts studying the crawlers. We ate cookies and drank cider, figured out who knew whom and how, and patted ourselves on the back for having organized ourselves into a play group *and* for having gotten ourselves dressed and out of the house.

When our babies started to walk, we ate fewer cookies, shadowed them everywhere, discussed haircuts, teething, and weaning. Our kids are now four plus. We leave them to play among themselves, watching from the corners of our eyes, intervening when necessary. We talk about nursery schools, and movies we've been to. We know each others' children practically as well as our own. Our bonds are deep, forged during both the toughest and the most joyful time of our lives.

Here are the reasons we think babies profit from a play group, not all of which will become manifest in the first year:

➤ They'll make their first friends.

➤ They'll be exposed to different toys in different households.

➤ They'll start getting accustomed to being in a group. By the time they hit day care, nursery school, or kindergarten, they'll already have a handle on interacting with other children.

➤ They'll become comfortable in the presence and care of other adults who are neither sitters nor relatives and take direction from them.

➤ They're provided with a safe emotional environment in which to move away from their own parent.

➤ Their sense of time begins to develop as they realize that play group is a regular event.

Our kids, all exceptional, of course, went through a staggering number of phases in relation to the group. Some glued themselves to their moms' legs. Others came alive when the group came to their homes. Some spent months observing the others from afar. Some managed to find and take apart every toy in the house. We were tolerant . . . to a point, which is important to the success of a play group. Understand that kids play differently. If your little one has her fun by watching from your lap, relax. No one can be the life of the party all the time.

LOIS: _Annie's doting aunts and grandmothers couldn't believe their eyes at her first-birthday party. Never had they seen such little babies (most of them from our play group) get along so well together, they clucked. Clearly these kids were already old friends._

THE NUTS AND BOLTS

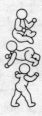 Are you sold? Following are some suggestions to keep in mind as you start up your own group. Most are based on our own experiences; some come from friends and friends of friends. Think about your own needs and create your group to fit (don't be too particular or you won't find cohorts). Cover as many bases as you can right when your group gets started, but don't expect the original parameters to stay the same. (Ours has evolved over the years we've been meeting.) Respect one another's preferences, handle problems as they come up, and be supportive, understanding, and flexible with one another.

First, think about who will comprise your group:

➤ You can limit _the adults_ to moms or dads, include sitters or not, and invite visiting relatives or not. Our group was generally just moms, although we were flexible; on occasion a dad or a sitter would bring one of the kids. Some groups are set up so that both parents attend, either together or on an alternating schedule of moms one week and dads the next. Some are for sitters only. You'll have a better time if all the adults share fundamental values about life and child rearing or can, at least, tolerate and respect one another's differences. Aim for *geographic proximity* so that getting together does not become an ordeal.

➤ As far as the babies are concerned, we recommend a maximum *age spread* of four to six months. With the exception of Kara, who is younger, our kids are all within four months of age. Since we started meeting when they were about six months old, the developmental differences were not as great as they would have been if we'd gotten them together much earlier.

➤ The ideal *number of kids* is between four and seven (ours was seven), bearing in mind that at least one baby probably won't make it each week. With fewer than four, you have more of a standing play date; more than seven and you might as well invite the Ringling Brothers. As far as *sex* goes, having the group evenly balanced between boys and girls at this age is nice but hardly necessary.

➤ Choose a *time* that works for everyone and stick to it until it no longer works for everyone. We've adjusted our starting hour a couple of times as nap times changed. But don't be too exact about starting and ending times.

➤ Limit the *length* to about two hours. That's long enough to give the babies the time they need to warm up and get comfortable and short enough that they won't get too revved up and turn cranky. We always try to break up while the kids are all still having fun, so that their goodbyes aren't tearful and they look forward to meeting again the next week.

Regarding location, you can consider the following options:

➤ Rotating homes gives you and your baby a variety of glimpses of others' ways of handling life with a baby. Your meeting will never be affected by weather; a bathroom and food supply are nearby; and the adults will have a place to sit down (aahh) and chat. (This is what we do, although we've never developed a rotation order, instead choosing where we meet each week depending on who's around, who's got evening plans, and so on.)

➤ On the other hand, you could always meet in the same house. If one group member has a fabulous recreation room or backyard and doesn't mind, this might be the way to go. Other members can balance the host's contribution by supplying the snacks, handling the cleanup, baby-sitting, or promising to put up visiting in-laws.

➤ Use a community space, if there's one available. Each member can bring juice and/or snacks (if permitted), or one member can cater each week on a rotating basis. Everyone shares cleanup, or one member does it each week on rotation. No fuss, no muss.

➤ Go places such as the aquarium, a museum, or elsewhere (see Chapter 3, "Out and About," for other possible destinations).

➤ Get together in the park or playground. (We did this once in a while when it was too gorgeous to be inside.) The down side is that once the babies are off and crawling, the adults don't get much of a visit since they'll be trailing their babies in every different direction.

LOIS: _A playground, being a public place, can also lead to sticky social situations. Annie once kept gravitating to a play group of like-aged kids and wanted to play alongside them. The mothers politely but coolly separated their sandbox toys from Annie's and talked past me. Neither of us had much fun. Even if you and your baby are part of a group, remember your manners._

Some of the sticky wickets we confronted or have heard of include:

➤ Baby-sitting: decide whether you want your group to double as a regular baby-sitting arrangement, enabling one or two of the adults to drop off their children and disappear for an hour or two. If not, will the group occasionally pinch hit? Define "occasionally" if you fear abuse. Or do you always want the group to maintain a one-on-one adult-to-baby ratio? We opted for the occasional pinch hit, which sometimes meant as little as fifteen minutes to walk the dog and sometimes meant extra time after play group when someone had an appointment.

➤ Snacktime: some groups make snacktime an important part of being together, while others don't want the hassle of buying, setting it up, or cleaning up after. Keep snacks simple, not too messy, and nutritious. One group we know of fell into the trap of competing with elaborate treats until their play group turned into a gourmet extravaganza fraught with all the tensions of a Cordon Bleu bake-off. Keep some baby-appropriate foods on hand (cheese, yogurt, fruit, for example) in case one of your pint-sized guests wasn't hungry at lunch and needs to raid the refrigerator. Have enough of each snack for the whole group.

➤ Bottle and food sharing: some parents don't mind if their babies share bottles and cups; others do. You'll probably skip the issue entirely if you keep food and drinks on a table or otherwise out of reach.

➤ Physical contact: some parents are concerned about the germs that spread when babies kiss, put one another's hands in their mouths, and the like. Establish a general rule and follow it.

T I P ➤ If you're invited into a group but don't like one of its aspects, you would do best not to join. (Some parents see red flags in disposable diapers, nonrecyclable plastic cups or plates, meat eating, and so on.) If you decide to join anyway, don't proselytize or be judgmental.

WAR AND PEACE

 If the babies in your group are tiny, you may be inclined to skip this part. Your little angels would never argue, grab, hit, or act up. Ha! As soon as they become mobile enough to get near each other, problems will arise.

Toy snatching is at the root of many arguments between babies. This sort of grabbing is usually one baby's expression of her momentary interest in something another baby has. At this age, it's strictly a matter of impulse, not a mean or willful act. Nonetheless, you needn't, and shouldn't, let it go unnoticed—impossible if one child is wailing, empty-handed. Gently but firmly wrest the stolen goods away and return the toy to the other child saying, "She had it first." Most little babies are easily distracted with another toy or game or a quick change of scenery. Next year you can introduce the idea of sharing by way of trading and taking turns.

Although more common after the first year, some younger-than-one babies, when they're upset or frustrated, hit or bite. Many parents are at a disciplinary loss when their child is the aggressor. Of the many ways to handle such transgressions, we've found a few most effective:

➤ If your child hits, take her hand slowly and firmly and say no in your most serious tone. (If you grab her hand angrily, you're sending her a mixed message: you verbally convey "no rough stuff" but your actions contradict your words.) When you let go, if her hand moves toward the other child, hold her hand and say no again. If biting is the problem, close her mouth with your hand and say, "You may not bite." Repeat as many times as necessary.

➤ After several times, remove your child from the situation for a short period. (This is what's known as a time-out, a tactic that will be more effective in the years to come; it can't hurt to get started now.) If your child's behavior persists once she rejoins the others, leave, explaining to her simply, "Because you won't stop biting, we can't play anymore."

➤ If one baby is causing the problem and the parent does not seem to be responding appropriately, the other adults should discuss it with the parent of the misbehaving child in as friendly and supportive tones as they can muster. The adult who neglects to guide an overspirited child needs to see the light. Remember that your own sweet pea may go through a Cujo phase next.

T I P ➤ Once in a while, hire baby-sitters, dress up, go out together to a nice restaurant, and spend the evening talking about anything but your kids! It took us about a year before we actually made it out one night. We barely recognized one another in our spotless dress-up clothes. What interesting conversations we had! In complete sentences.

We wish you as much pleasure from your play dates and play group as we have had from ours. There is nothing more thrilling, with the exception of witnessing your own child's development, than watching the personalities of several wonderful children blossom—kids you've known since their babyhood and for whom you feel genuine affection. If you manage to keep your group going for some time, you will also reap the profound pleasure of seeing your child's attachments to her first friends deepen. And who knows what may come of the friendships you make with the other parents? Maybe you'll write a book of your own.

PART

III

Appendices

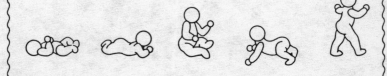

APPENDIX A

Words to Songs

It doesn't matter if you know the "right" tune for these songs. Many of them are merely rhymes that you can sing or chant in any old singsong way. If you see numbers above the lyrics, that means you can play the tune on a typical eight-note toy xylophone. Number 1 corresponds to the lowest note, which is the longest bar, equivalent to middle C on a piano.

GENERAL NURSERY RHYMES

BAA, BAA, BLACK SHEEP

```
1   1   5   5   6   6   6 6 5
Baa, baa, black sheep, have you any wool?
```

```
4   4   3   3   2   2   1
Yes sir, yes sir, three bags full.
```

```
5   5   5   4   4   4   3   3   3   2
One for my master and one for my dame.
```

```
5   5   5   4 4 4       4   3   3   3   2
One for the little boy [girl] who lives down the lane.
```

```
1   1   5   5   6   6   6 6 5
Baa, baa, black sheep, have you any wool?
```

```
4   4   3   3   2   2   1
Yes sir, yes sir, three bags full.
```

173

RAIN, RAIN, GO AWAY
Rain, rain, go away,
Come again another day.
Little Johnny wants to play.

RUB A DUB DUB
Rub a dub dub, three men in a tub.
Who do you think they be?
The butcher, the baker, the candlestick maker.
Turn them out, knaves all three.

JACK AND JILL
Jack and Jill went up the hill
To fetch a pail of water.
Jack fell down and broke his crown
And Jill came tumbling after.

MARY HAD A LITTLE LAMB
(chorus)

3 2 1   2 3 3   3   2 2 2   3 5 5
Mary had a little lamb, little lamb, little lamb.

3 2 1   2 3 3   3   3   2   2   3   2 1
Mary had a little lamb, whose fleece was white as snow.

(verses, repeat chorus after each one)
It followed her to school one day, school one day, school one day.
It followed her to school one day, which was against the rules.

It made the children laugh and play, laugh and play, laugh and play.
It made the children laugh and play to see a lamb at school.

Why does the lamb love Mary so, love Mary so, love Mary so?
Why does the lamb love Mary so, the eager children cried.

Cause Mary loves the lamb you know, lamb you know, lamb you
    know.
Cause Mary loves the lamb you know, the teacher did reply.

JACK BE NIMBLE
Jack be nimble
Jack be quick
Jack jumped over the candlestick.

LITTLE BOY BLUE
Little Boy Blue come blow your horn.
The sheep's in the meadow, the cow's in the corn.
Where is the boy who looks after the sheep?
He's under a haystack fast asleep.

Will you wake him?
No, not I.
For if I do,
He'll surely cry.

LITTLE MISS MUFFET
Little Miss Muffet sat on her tuffet
Eating her curds and whey.
Along came a spider who sat down beside her
And frightened Miss Muffet away.

WEE WILLIE WINKIE
Wee Willie Winkie runs through the town.
Upstairs and downstairs, in his nightgown.
Rapping at the window, crying at the lock.
Are the children in their beds?
For now it's eight o'clock.

GEORGIE PORGIE
Georgie Porgie pudding and pie
Kissed the girls and made them cry.
When the boys came out to play
Georgie Porgie ran away.

GRAND OLD DUKE OF YORK

6   5   4   4 1   1 4   4 5 5 2   2   5
Oh, the grand old Duke of York, he had ten thousand men

4 3   3   3 3 3 3   3 3 3   3 2 1   1
He marched them up to the top of the hill and he marched them

   2   3 4
down again.

6   4   4   4   1 1   1   4   4   5   5   5
And when they were up, they were up. And when they were

   2   2   2   5
down they were down.

4   3   3   3   3 3 3 3   3 3   2   1   1 2 3
And when they were only halfway up, they were neither up nor

   4
down.

SEE SAW, MARGERY DAW
See saw, Margery Daw
Jackie shall have a new master.
He shall earn but a penny a day,
Because he can't work any faster.

BOUNCING RHYMES

RIDE A COCK HORSE
Ride a cock horse to Banbury Cross
To see a fine lady upon a white horse.
Rings on her fingers and bells on her toes,
She shall have music wherever she goes.

TO MARKET, TO MARKET
To market, to market to buy a fat pig
Home again, home again, jiggedy jig.
To market, to market to buy a fat hog.
Home again, home again, jiggedy jog.
To market, to market to buy a plum bun.
Home again, home again, market is done.

THIS IS THE WAY MY BABY RIDES
This is the way my baby rides,
My baby rides,
My baby rides,
This is the way my baby rides,
So early in the morning.

JENNY O'FLYNN
Jenny O'Flynn and her old gray mare
Went off to see the country fair.
The bridge fell down *(open knees)*.
The mare fell in *(drop baby through knees and pick up again)*.
And that was the last of Jenny O'Flynn O'Flynn O'Flynn O'Flynn.

SHOE THE OLD HORSE
Shoe the old horse.
Shoe the old mare.
But let the little pony run
Bare bare bare.

TROT, TROT TO BOSTON
Trot, trot to Boston.
Trot, trot to Lynn.
Trot, trot home again.
We all fall in.

RIDE, BABY, RIDE
Ride, baby, ride. Chachachachachacha
Ride, that pony, ride. Chachachachachacha
Ride, baby, ride. Chachachachachacha
Whoooaaaa!

THIS IS THE WAY THE LADIES RIDE

This is the way the ladies ride *(gentle bounce)*.
gobbity gobbity gobbity
This is the way the gentlemen ride *(bigger bounce)*.
gobbity gobbity gobbity
This is the way the farmers ride *(lift one heel at a time for trot)*.
gobbity gobbity gobbity
This is the way the hunters ride *(biggest bounce)*.
gobbity gobbit gobbity
Till they fall in a ditch with a FLOP *(drop the baby gently between your knees)*.

MAMA AND PAPA AND UNCLE JOHN

Mama and Papa and Uncle John
Went to town one by one.
Mama fell off *(lean to left)*.
And Papa fell off *(lean to right)*.
But Uncle John went on and on and on and on *(bouncing)*.

LONDON BRIDGE

5   6   5   4 3 4   5   2 3   4   3 4   5
London Bridge is falling down, falling down, falling down *(put baby on your ankle or knee and bounce with each falling down)*

5   6   5   4 3 4   5   2 5   3 1
London Bridge is falling down, my fair lady [or laddy].

Build it up with iron bars, iron bars, iron bars
Build it up with iron bars, my fair lady.

Build it up with silver and gold, silver and gold, silver and gold
Build it up with silver and gold, my fair lady.

Take the key and lock her up, lock her up, lock her up,
Take the key and lock her up, my fair lady.

LITTLE RED WAGON
(chorus)
Bumping up and down in my little red wagon
Bumping up and down in my little red wagon
Bumping up and down in my little red wagon
Won't you be my darlin'?

(verses, repeat chorus after each one)
One wheel's off and the axle's broken *(repeat twice more)*.
Won't you be my darlin'?

(Child's name) is going to fix it with his *(name a tool)* *(repeat twice more)*
Won't you be my darlin'? *(repeat using different names and tools)*

Hands and Feet, Fingers and Toes

EENSY WEENSY SPIDER *(itsy bitsy, eensy weensy . . . whatever)*
The eensy weensy spider climbed up the water spout.
Down came the rain and washed the spider out.
Out came the sun and dried up all the rain.
And the eensy weensy spider climbed up the spout again.

   Variation: Using a booming voice, repeat the song using "the great big spider" and this time place the fingertips of your left hand atop the fingertips of your right hand and pump them. Using a teeny-tiny voice, sing the song about a teeny-tiny spider.

ROUND AND ROUND THE GARDEN
Round and round the garden *(walk your fingers around the baby's palm or tummy)*
Runs the teddy bear.
One step, two steps *(walk fingers toward chin)*
And tickle him under there.

COME AND LOOKASEE
Come and lookasee, here is my mama *(thumb)*.
Come and lookasee, here is my papa *(pointer)*.
Come and lookasee, brother so tall *(index)*
Sister *(ring finger)*, baby *(littlest finger)*, I love them all! *(kiss the baby's hand)*

THIS LITTLE PIGGY
   Curl baby's fingers into a fist or open a fist finger by finger with:

This little piggy went to market.
This little piggy stayed home.
This little piggy had roast beef.
This little piggy had none.
And this little piggy went
Wee, wee, wee, all the way home.

or

This little baby rocked the cradle.
This little baby jumped in bed.
This little baby crawled all over.
This little baby bumped his head.
This little baby played hide and seek.
Where did all the babies go? Let's PEEK!

THESE ARE MY BABY'S FINGERS
These are my baby's fingers.
These are my baby's toes.
This is my baby's belly button.
Around and around it goes *(tickle tummy)*.

TEN LITTLE FINGERS
   Make the corresponding motions as you say this rhyme:

I have ten little fingers and they all belong to me.
I can make them do things,
Would you like to see?
I can close them up tight,

I can open them wide,
I can hold them up high,
I can hold them down low,
I can wave them to and fro,
And I can hold them just so.

TEN LITTLE INDIANS

4   4 4   4   4 4   6   8 8   6 5 4
One little, two little, three little Indians.

5   5 5   5   5 5   3   5 5   3 2 1
Four little, five little, six little Indians.

4 4   4 4   4   4 4   6   8 8   6 5 4
Seven little, eight little, nine little Indians.

5   5 5   1 2 3   4
Ten little Indian boys (or girls).

WHERE IS THUMBKIN?
    Hide hands behind your back and sing to the tune of "Frère Jacques":

Where is Thumbkin?
Where is Thumbkin? Here I am *(bring one fist out and raise your
        thumb)*!
Here I am *(out comes the other)*!
How are you today, sir *(bow one thumb to the other)*?
Very well, I thank you *(bow the other thumb)*.
Run away *(bring one hand back behind your back)*.
Run away *(bring the other hand behind your back)*.

    Repeat using all the fingers: pointer, tall man, ring man, and
pinkie.

THE TURTLE
I have a little turtle who lives in the sand.
He swims down in the water *(make swimming motions with your hands)*
And crawls on the land *(crawl your fingers up the baby's leg)*.
He snapped at a spider *(snap your fingers)*
He snapped at a flea *(snap again)*
He snapped at a minnow *(once more)*
And he snapped at me *(last time)*.
He caught the spider *(clap)*
He caught the flea *(clap again)*
He caught the minnow *(last clap)*
But he couldn't catch me.

TWO LITTLE BLUEBIRDS
Two little bluebirds sitting on a hill.
One named Jack *(hold up one index finger)*.
The other named Jill *(hold up the other index finger)*.
Fly away, Jack *(one hand disappears behind you)*
Fly away, Jill *(the other hand disappears)*.
Come back, Jack *(hand reappears)*.
Come back, Jill *(other hand reappears)*.

BINGO
There was a farmer had a dog and Bingo was his name, oh.
B-I-N-G-O
B-I-N-G-O
B-I-N-G-O
And Bingo was his name, oh.

Repeat, replacing one letter (starting with the *b*) with a clap each time until, for the last verse, the dog's name is entirely claps.

FIVE LITTLE MONKEYS
Five little monkeys jumping on the bed *(bounce all five fingers of one hand on the open palm of the other)*
One fell off and bumped his head *(rub your head)*
Mama called the doctor *(dial phone)*
And the doctor said, "No more monkeys jumping on the bed!" *(wag index finger in disapproval)*

OPEN, SHUT THEM
(Start with closed fists)
Open, shut them *(open fists, spread fingers, close both fists)*.
Open, shut them *(ditto)*.
Give a little clap, clap, clap *(clap three times)*.
Open, shut them *(open, spread, and close again)*.
Open, shut them *(ditto)*.
Put them in your lap *(put hands in lap)*.
Creep them, crawl them, creep them, crawl them *(walk fingers up tummy, chest, and neck)*.
Right up to your chin, chin, chin *(tap the baby's chin three times)*
Open wide your little mouth,
But do not let them in *(quickly move hands away)*.

THIS OLD MAN
(Clap or knock when you sing the knick-knacks)

5   3   5   5 3   5
This old man, he played one

6 5   4   3   2 3 4
He played knick-knack on my thumb

3   4 5   1   1 1 1   1   2   3   4 5
With a knick-knack paddy-whack, give the dog a bone,

5   2   2   4   3 2   1
This old man came rolling home.

Repeat with these rhymes: two, shoe; three, knee; four, door; five, hive; six, sticks; seven, up to heaven; eight, gate; nine, spine; ten, once again.

POP! GOES THE WEASEL
Teach the baby to clap or throw up his arms at the POP!

1 1 2   2   3 5 3   1   1   1   1   2   4   3   1
All around the cobbler's bench, the monkey chased the weasel.

1   1 1 2   2   3 5 3 1 6   2   4   3   1
The monkey thought 'twas all in fun. POP! goes the weasel.

5 8 8 6 6 7   7 5   5 8 8 6 6 7 5
A penny for a spool of thread, a penny for a needle.

4   3   4   5   6   7 8   6   2   4   3   1
That's the way the money goes, POP! goes the weasel.

BODY GAMES

PAT-A-CAKE
Pat-a-cake *(clap)*
Pat-a-cake *(clap)*
Baker's man *(clap)*.
Bake me *(clap)* a cake *(clap)* as fast *(clap)* as you can *(clap)*.
Pat it *(make patting motions)*, and prick it *(poke baby's tummy)*,
And mark it with a *B (draw letter on baby's tummy)*.
And put it in the oven *(slide your hands toward baby and tickle him)*
For baby *(point to baby)* and me *(point to yourself)*.

HICKORY, DICKORY, DOCK

3   45 4   32 3
Hickory, dickory, dock,

3 3   5 4 2 3
The mouse ran up the clock *(walk your fingers up the baby's body)*.

3 3 3   5
The clock struck one *(tap the baby once on the nose or forehead)*,

5 4   4 6
The mouse ran down *(walk your fingers back down the baby's body)*,

```
5    65   4    32   1
```
Hickory, dickory, dock.

ROW, ROW, ROW YOUR BOAT

```
1    1    1    2    3    3 2   3    4    5
```
Row, row, row your boat, gently down the stream *(row the baby's arms)*.

```
8    88   5    55   3    33   1    11   5    4    3    2 1
```
Merrily, merrily, merrily, merrily, life is but a dream.

I'M A LITTLE TEAPOT

```
1    23 4  5    8
```
I'm a little teapot *(hold the baby's hands at his sides)*

```
6    8    5
```
Short and stout.

```
4    4 4  3    3
```
Here is my handle *(bend one arm so his hand is on his hip)*,

```
2    2 2  1
```
Here is my spout *(hold his other arm out)*.

```
1    23   4    5         8 6   8    5
```
When I get all steamed up hear me SHOUT *(loud)*!

```
5    8    6    5 4 4  3    2    1
```
Just tip me over and pour me out *(tip him over)*.

IF YOU'RE HAPPY AND YOU KNOW IT
If you're happy and you know it clap your hands *(clap clap)*.
If you're happy and you know it clap your hands *(clap clap)*.
If you're happy and you know it and you really want to show it
If you're happy and you know it clap your hands *(clap clap)*.

Substitute any action or direction your baby can do such as: shake your head, kick your feet, wave bye-bye, touch your nose, blow a kiss, stick out your tongue.

CHIN CHOPPER
(Use a gentle touch or this game won't be any fun at all)
Knock on the door *(use your knuckles on the baby's forehead)*.
Peep in *(lift one of baby's eyelids)*.
Open the latch *(press the tip of the baby's nose up)*.
And walk in *(walk two fingers on the baby's bottom lip)*.
Chin chopper, chin chopper, chin chopper chin *(using your thumb
    and forefinger, raise and lower the baby's bottom jaw)*.
Chin chopper, chin chopper, chin chopper chin *(repeat)*.

THE WHEELS ON THE BUS

1   4   4 4 4 6 8   6 4
The wheels on the bus go round and round *(roll your hands like a
    paddle wheel)*,

5   3 1   8   6 4
Round and round, round and round *(keep rolling)*.

1   4   4 4 4 6 8   6 4
The wheels on the bus go round and round *(keep it up)*

5 11 4
All over town.

For additional verses, sing about the things that happen on the bus and make appropriate motions: the driver says move on back *(jerk your thumb over your shoulder)*; the lights go blink *(make a fist, then open and shut your fingers)*; doors open and close *(put your palms together, open and close them)*; people go up and down *(bounce the baby)*; wipers go swish swish swish *(move hands back and forth)*; babies say wah wah wah; moms and dads say I love you.

HOKEY POKEY
You put your right arm in *(move his arm)*.
You take your right arm out *(ditto)*.
You put your right arm in *(ditto)*.
And you shake it all about *(shake his arm gently)*.

You do the Hokey Pokey *(hold his fists and wiggle them simultaneously).*
And you turn yourself around *(pick up the baby and spin around
   with him).*
That's what it's all about.

SKINNAMARINK
   (Do whatever hand motions you like during the skinnamarinky
dinky doo part)

Skinnamarinky dinky dink, skinnamarinky doo
I love you *(point to your eye, cross your hands over your heart, point
   to baby)*
Skinnamarinky dinky dink, skinnamarinky doo
I love you *(point to your eye, cross your hands over your heart, point
   to baby)*
I love you in the morning and in the afternoon *(make a cradle of
   your arms and rock imaginary baby)*
I love you in the evening underneath the moon *(raise your arms
   and make a moon in the sky with your hands)*
Skinnamarinky dinky dink, skinnamarinky doo
I love you *(point to your eye, cross your hands over your heart, point
   to baby)*

HANDS ON SHOULDERS
Hands on shoulders, hands on knees,
Put them behind you, if you please.
Touch your shoulders, now your nose,
Now your hair, and now your toes.
Put your hands up high in the air,
Down at your sides, and touch your hair.
Hands up high as before
Now clap your hands, one, two, three, four.

HEAD, SHOULDERS, KNEES, AND TOES
(Touch the baby's head, shoulders, knees, and toes, or guide his hands so he can do it himself as you sing this song.)

Head, shoulders, knees, and toes, knees and toes.
Head, shoulders, knees, and toes, knees and toes.
Eyes and ears and mouth and nose.
Head, shoulders, knees, and toes, knees and toes.

RING AROUND THE ROSIE
(For at least two walkers and their grown-ups)

Ring around the rosie *(hold hands and walk in a circle)*.
A pocket full of posies *(keep going)*.
Ashes, ashes, all fall down *(collapse on the floor)*!

The cows are in the meadow eating buttercups *(pat the floor with your hands)*
Thunder *(pound the floor)*!
Lightning *(make lightning bolts with your fingers)*!
All jump up *(stand up)*!

Animal and Other Funny Noise Songs

OLD MACDONALD

4   4   4   1   2   2 1   6 6 5 5 4
Old MacDonald had a farm, E-I-E-I-O.

1   4   4   4   1   2   2 1   6 6 5 5 4
And on that farm he had a _____ E-I-E-I-O.

1   1 4   4   4   1   1 4   4   4
With a _____ _____ here and a _____ _____ there.

4   4 4   4   4 4   4   4 4   4 4
Here a _____, there a _____, everywhere a _____

    4

    _____ .

4   4   4   1   2   2 1   6 6 5 5 4
Old MacDonald had a farm, E-I-E-I-O.

cows moo, pigs oink, ducks quack, sheep baa, geese honk, horses neigh, fish glub, frogs croak, kangaroos boing, etc.

CAMPTOWN RACES

5   5   5   3 5   6   5   3   3   2   3   2
The Camptown ladies sing their song, doo-dah, doo-dah

5   5   3   5   6   5   3   2   3   2   1
Camptown racetrack's five miles long, oh, doo-dah-day.

5   5   5   3   5 6   5   3   3   2   3   2
Oh, see those horses round the bend, doo-dah, doo-dah.

5   5   3   5   6 5 3   2   3   2   1
Guess that race will never end, oh, doo-dah day.

(chorus)

1 1 1 3   5   8   6 6 6 8   6 5
Goin' to run all night, goin' to run all day.

5 5   5   3   3 5 5 6   5 3   2   3   4 3   2 2 1
I'll bet my money on a bobtail nag, somebody bet on the bay.

The long-tail filly and the big black horse, doo-dah, doo-dah.
They fly the track and they both cut across, oh, doo-dah-day.
The blind horse stickin' in a big mud hole, doo-dah, doo-dah.
Can't touch bottom with a ten-foot pole, oh, doo-dah-day.

(repeat chorus)

THERE WAS AN OLD LADY WHO SWALLOWED A FLY
There was an old lady who swallowed a fly,
I don't know why she swallowed a fly,
Perhaps she'll die *(cry)*.

There was an old lady who swallowed a spider,
That wiggled and jiggled and tickled inside her *(tickle baby)*.
She swallowed the spider to catch the fly.
I don't know why she swallowed the fly.
Perhaps she'll die.

   Other verses:

swallowed a bird, how absurd, she swallowed a bird.
swallowed a cat, how about that, she swallowed a cat.
swallowed a dog, my what a hog, she swallowed a dog.
swallowed a goat, got stuck in her throat, she swallowed a goat.
swallowed a cow, I don't know how she swallowed a cow.
swallowed a horse, she died of course.

OVER IN THE MEADOW
Over in the meadow (in the sand in the sun)
Lived an old mother (turtle) and her little (turtle one).
(Dig) said the mother. We (dig) said the (one).
So they (dug) all day in the (sand in the sun).

   For other verses, replace the words in parentheses with:

Where the stream runs blue, fish, fishes two, swim, swim, two,
     swam, stream so blue.
In a hole in a tree, owl, owls three, sleep, sleep, three, slept, hole
     in the tree.
By the old barn door, mousie, mousies four, squeak, squeak, four,
     squeaked, by the old barn door.
In a snug beehive, bee, bees five, buzz, buzz, five, buzzed, snug
     beehive.
In a nest built of sticks, crow, crows six, caw, caw, six, cawed,
     nest built of sticks.

Where the grass grows even, frog, frogs seven, jump, jump, seven,
    jumped, where the grass grows even.
By the old mossy gate, lizard, lizards eight, bask, bask, eight,
    basked, mossy gate.
By the big scotch pine, duck, ducks nine, quack, quack, nine,
    quacked, by the big scotch pine.
In a cozy wee den, beaver, beavers ten, gnaw, gnaw, ten, gnawed
    cozy wee den.

ANIMAL FAIR

3 5   5 5 6 6 3 5
I went to the animal fair.

3 5   5 5 6   3   4
The birds and the beasts were there.

5 7 7 7   6 6 7   7 7 7
The big baboon, by the light of the moon,

6 5   5 5 6 3   5
Was combing his auburn hair.

3 5   5 5   6   3   5
You ought to have seen the monk.

3 5   5 5 6 63   4
He jumped on the elephant's trunk.

5 7 7 7   7   6 7 7 7 7
The elephant sneezed and fell on his knees

6 5   5   5   5 6 7 8   1 1   1 1   1
And that was the end of the monk, the monk, the monk, the

1
monk?

CANNIBAL KING
The cannibal king with the big nose ring
Fell in love with the dusty maid.
And every night by the pale moonlight
Across the lake he swam.

(chorus)
Ba-room, ba-room, ba-room ba-dee-a-dee-yay
Ba-room, ba-room, ba-room ba-dee-a-dee-yay.

He hugged and he kissed his pretty little miss
In the shade of the bamboo tree.
And every night by the pale moonlight
This is what I heard him say.

(repeat chorus)

We'll build a bungalow big enough for two
Big enough for two my darling, big enough for two.
And when we're married happy we'll be
Under the bamboo, under the bamboo tree.

TINGALAYO
(chorus)

3 5 6 5 4   4 4 5 4   3
Tingalayo, run little donkey, run.

3 5 6 5 4   4 4 3 2   1
Tingalayo, run little donkey, run.

(verses, repeat chorus after each one)

5 8 7   6   4 7 6   5
My donkey walks, my donkey talks

3 6 5   4   4   4 5   4   3
My donkey eats with a knife and fork.

3 8 7   6   6 7 6   5
My donkey walks, my donkey talks

3   6   5   4   4   4 3   2   1
My donkey eats with a knife and fork.

My donkey eats, my donkey sleeps,
My donkey kicks with his two hind feet.
My donkey eats, my donkey sleeps,
My donkey kicks with his two hind feet.

My donkey hee, my donkey haw,
My donkey sleeps in a bed of straw.
My donkey hee, my donkey haw.
My donkey sleeps in a bed of straw.

Lullabies

TWINKLE, TWINKLE, LITTLE STAR
(chorus) (same tune for the alphabet song)

1   1   5   5 6 6   5   4   4 3   3   2   2   1
Twinkle, twinkle little star, how I wonder what you are.

5   5 4   4   3   3 2   5   5 4   4   3 3   2
Up above the world so high, like a diamond in the sky.

1   1   5   5 6 6   5   4   4 3   3   2   2   1
Twinkle, twinkle little star, how I wonder what you are.

Verses (repeat chorus after each):
When the blazing sun is gone, when he nothing shines upon,
Then you show your little light, twinkle, twinkle all the night . . .

In the dark blue sky you keep and often through my curtains peep,
for you never shut your eye, till the sun is in the sky . . .

As your bright and tiny spark, lights the traveler in the dark,
Though I know not what you are, twinkle, twinkle little star . . .

When the traveler in the dark thanks you for your tiny spark,
He could not see which way to go, if you did not twinkle so . . .

ROCK-A-BYE BABY

Rock-a-bye baby on the tree top.
When the wind blows, the cradle will rock.
When the bough breaks, the cradle will fall.
And down will come baby, cradle and all.

SLEEP, BABY, SLEEP

Sleep, baby, sleep.
Thy father guards the sheep.
Thy mother shakes the dreamland tree,
And down fall pleasant dreams for thee,
Sleep, baby, sleep.
Sleep, baby, sleep.

LULLABY AND GOOD NIGHT

3 3 5 3   3   5   3 5 8 7 6 6 5
Lullaby and good night, with roses bedight,

 2 3 4   223 4   24 7 6 5   7   8
With down over spread is Baby's wee bed.

1   1   8   6   4   5   3   1   4   5   6 5
Lay thee down now and rest, may thy slumbers be blest.

1   1   8   6   4   5   3   1   4   3   2 1
Lay thee down now and rest, may thy slumbers be blest.

or

Lullaby and good night
In the sky stars are bright.
Round your head, flowers gay,
Scent your slumbers till day.
Close your eyes now and rest,
May these hours be blest.

HE'S GOT THE WHOLE WORLD IN HIS HANDS
He's got the whole world in His hands
He's got the whole world in His hands
He's got the whole world in His hands
He's got the whole world in His hands.

He's got the little bitty baby in His hands
He's got the little bitty baby in His hands
He's got the little bitty baby in His hands
He's got the whole world in His hands.

HUSH, LITTLE BABY

2   7 7 7 8 6 6 6 6
Hush, little baby, don't say a word.

2 2   6 6 6 6 7 6 5 5
Mama's (or Papa's) gonna buy you a mockingbird.

2 2 7 7 8 7 6 6
And if that (mocking bird don't sing),

2 2 6 6 6 6 7 6 5 5
Mama's gonna buy you a (diamond ring).

Other verses: diamond ring turns brass, looking glass; looking
glass gets broke, billy goat; billy goat don't pull, cart and bull; cart
and bull turns over, dog named Rover; dog named Rover don't
bark, horse and cart; horse and cart falls down, you'll still be the
sweetest little baby in town.

KUMBAYA

1 3 5 5 5   6 6 5
Kumbaya, my Lord, kumbaya,

1 3 5 5 5   4 3 2
Kumbaya, my Lord, kumbaya,

1 3 5 5 5   6 6 5
Kumbaya, my Lord, kumbaya,

4 3 1 2   2 1
Oh, Lord, kumbaya.

Other verses:

someone's singing, Lord, Kumbaya *(repeat)*;
someone's dancing, Lord, Kumbaya;
someone's crying, Lord, Kumbaya;
Come by here, Lord, Kumbaya.

TAPS

1 1 4 1   4 6
Day is done gone the sun.

1   4 6   1   4 6   1   4 6
From the lake, from the hills, from the sky.

4 6 8   6 4 1
All is well, safely rest.

1   1 4
God is nigh.

AMAZING GRACE

1　4 654　6　　5　　4　　　2　1
Amazing grace how sweet the sound

1　　4　65 4　6　　　58　8
That saved a wretch like me.

68　8　 654 6　　5　　4　　2　1
Ionce was lost but now I'm found

1　4　　654 6　5 4
was blind, but now I see.

APPENDIX B

Mail Order Sources

FOR MUSIC

HearthSong, Box B, Sebastopol, CA 95473; (800) 325-2502.

Wireless, A Gift Catalog for Fans and Friends of Public Radio, Box 64422, St. Paul, MN 55164; (800) 669-9999.

Music for Little People, Box 1460, 1144 Redway Drive, Redway, CA 95560; (800) 346-4445.

Alcazar's Kiddie Catalogue, Box 429, Waterbury, VT 05676; (802) 244-8657.

Chinaberry Book Service, 2830 Via Orange Way, Suite 13, Spring Valley, CA 92078; (800) 777-5205.

Ladyslipper, Box 3130, Durham, NC 27705; (919) 683-1570.

A Gentle Wind, Box 3103, Albany, NY 12203; (518) 482-9023.

FOR VIDEO

Critic's Choice Video, Box 549, Elk Grove Village, IL 60009; (800) 367-7765.

Troll Learn & Play, 100 Corporate Dr., Mahwah, NJ 07498-1053; (800) 247-6106.

GENERAL PRODUCTS

Right Start, Right Start Plaza, 5334 Sterling Center Dr., Westlake Village, CA 91361; (800) 548-8531.

One Step Ahead, Box 517, Lake Bluff, IL 60044; (800) 274-8440.

FOR TOYS

HearthSong, Box B, Sebastopol, CA 95473; (800) 325-2502.

Lillian Vernon, 510 So. Fulton Avenue, Mt. Vernon, NY 10550; (914) 633-6300.

Childcraft, Box 29149, Mission, KS 66201; (800) 631-5657.

Sesame Street Catalog, Box 29166, Lenexa, KS 66201; (800) 367-8995.

The Great Kids Co., Box 609, Lewisville, NC 27023; (800) 533-2166.

Animal Town, Box 485, Healdsburg, CA 95448; (800) 445-8642.

Toys to Grow On, Box 17, Long Beach, CA 90801; (800) 542-8338.

Back to Basics Toys, 2707 Pittman Dr., Silver Spring, MD 20910; (800) 356-5360.

Sensational Beginnings, Box 2009, 300 Detroit, Suite E, Monroe, MI 48161; (800) 444-2147.

F. A. O. Schwarz, 767 Fifth Ave., New York, NY 10153; (800) 426-8697.

FOR BOOKS

Barnes & Noble, 1 Pond Rd., Rockleigh, NJ 07647; (800) 233-2470.

Chinaberry Book Service, 2780 Via Orange Way, Suite B, Spring Valley, CA 91978; (800) 776-2242.

Gryphon House Early Childhood Book Catalog, Box 275, Mount Rainier, MD 20712; (800) 638-0928.

HearthSong, Box B, Sebastopol, CA 95473; (800) 325-2502.

Play Fair Toys, 1690 28th Street, Boulder, CO 80301; (800) 824-7255.

Wireless, P.O. Box 64422, St. Paul, MN 55164; (800) 669-9999.

Just for Kids!, Box 29141, Shawnee, KS 66201; (800) 654-6963.

APPENDIX C

A Word on First Birthdays

A baby's first birthday is a tremendously significant event. She's grown from a completely helpless infant to a mobile and communicative, albeit small, person. And you've managed that first year more competently than you ever thought you could.

The thing to remember is that none of that emotional, sentimental stuff that makes her first birthday so important to you and the other adults in her life matters to her. Nor does it *have* to be celebrated with the biggest birthday bash in the history of babykind. This is not to say that she won't enjoy the party. She may have the time of her life. But will you?

Family styles differ as much as do babies' personalities. Some of us love to throw wild bashes. Some of us kept our parties small. If you opt for the big bash, be prepared for your baby to cling to your leg throughout the extravaganza, refusing to interact with any except the most familiar adults. However, she may also surprise you by playing happily with her friends on the floor while the adults look on with pride and joy.

LOIS: *I ignored every rule in every book when I planned Annie's party, inviting all of Annie's playmates and their parents, and every relative in driving distance, and all of our pre-Annie friends. It was a wonderful party.*

LIBBY: *I waited until the last minute, and Sam ended up with three miniparties: a play-group celebration, a gathering of our friends with children, and a relatives-only toast.*

But, whichever course you take, remember to consider the children's needs:

➤ Time the party so it doesn't conflict with her nap.

➤ Keep it short.

➤ Take most of the pictures early in the party before the kids get cranky . . . and grubby.

➤ Open the presents after the tiny guests have left if you think seeing others opening her gifts and playing with her new stuff will upset your child. Nine out of ten times, it will.

Here are some fun ideas for whatever size party you choose:

➤ Hire a favorite sitter or designate a relative to help out.

➤ Put the party hats on stuffed animals, not the real tykes.

➤ Break out some new toys.

➤ Play ring around the rosie.

➤ Sit all the babes on your biggest bed sheet, have the adults hold the edges, and slowly walk around in a circle to "Wheels on the Bus," bouncing them gently when you get to the "people on the bus go up and down" verse. "Little Red Wagon" is another good choice.

➤ If it's nice outside, have an outdoor bubble fest with one-on-one adult supervision.

➤ Sit the kids in a circle, give each a musical instrument, and let them accompany their own favorite song. Or teach them a new audience participation song like the "Hokey Pokey."

➤ Break up before the kids crash from the excitement and icing.

T I P ➤ Instead of buying standard party favors, most of which are inappropriate for children this age, give each tot a Golden Book, a sand toy, some sidewalk chalk, a small box of crayons (or a handful in a tiny shopping bag), a can of Play-Doh, or even a cute toothbrush. Buying a toy that comes as a large set and dividing it among the children often works out more cheaply.

If you're not up for inviting hordes of people to your home but nonetheless went to celebrate, there are other possibilities:

➤ Invite only a few of her pals (all or none from any given play group), not every other baby you know.

➤ Turn play group into a party by dressing the kids up a little and serving decorated cupcakes or a cake.

➤ Head for the zoo, a museum, or a boat show as a family or with one favorite playmate. This follows the old rule of thumb: one guest for every year.

➤ Set aside some time to look at the last twelve months in photos together. Who is that wrinkled baby?

➤ Start a tradition by taking a photograph of the birthday kid in a special place to which you can return each year.

➤ Celebrate the milestone by buying a "big kid" thing such as a cup, pair of shoes, or trike.

➤ Start a collection of something special such as music boxes or classic children's books that you can add to each year.

➤ Let the birthday baby lower her face into a cupcake, take a picture, and celebrate your successful first year of parenthood.

The Gift Horse

What's a birthday without presents? Keep these suggestions in mind when you're shopping for first-birthday gifts and when others call to ask what the baby would like. Some will be too advanced on the birthday itself; stash these and try them out later in the year. Make sure that any *really* inappropriate toys disappear instantly— especially those that can be swallowed or require one-on-one supervision.

TOYS

➤ big, fat crayons and sidewalk chalk

➤ Magna Doodle, by Tyco, a magnetic, mess-free drawing board

➤ wooden puzzles in which each piece has its own niche and a little peg for easy handling

➤ a shape sorter

➤ building blocks and other nesting and stacking toys

➤ large interlocking beads

➤ a pull toy

➤ a puppet (does the child have a favorite animal?)

➤ wheeled vehicles with passengers

➤ plastic tools

➤ kitchen equipment

➤ a ride-on or push toy

MUSIC

➤ a child's cassette player

➤ cassettes of favorite or classic stories (some have accompanying books)

➤ musical instruments

➤ song books with music

➤ music videos (see Chapter 6, "For a Song")

BOOKS

Any of the books mentioned in Chapter 7, "Book 'Em," for crawlers or cruisers, or any of the following, which they will enjoy in the coming year:

➤ alphabet books

➤ counting books

➤ books about colors

➤ pop-up books

➤ poetry anthologies (Shel Silverstein writes funny ones)

➤ books of activities that she'll be able to do (with an adult, probably) this year

➤ anything by Dr. Seuss

➤ a volume or two of beautifully illustrated fairy tales to be set aside for the years to come or as heirlooms

Of the many wonderful books and series to choose from, these were among our kids' favorites.

➤ *Max's Breakfast* by Rosemary Wells (New York: Very First Books, Dial Books for Young Readers, 1985; also in the series *Max's Bath, Max's Bedtime, Max's Birthday,* and others); the sassy, contrary bunny Max is Everytoddler.

➤ *My First Look at Clothes*, a Dorling Kindersley Book (New York: Random House, 1991; also in the series: *My First Look at Sizes, Colors, Noises, Things that Go,* and others); a large-format book with engaging photographs organized to invite comparisons and discussion. These came out when our kids turned two, but they're great for one-year-olds.

➤ *Richard Scarry's Best Word Book Ever* by Richard Scarry (Racine, Wisc.: A Golden Book, Western Publishing Co., Inc., 1980); each page is a busy tumble of Scarry's endearing little creatures engaged in activities that interest toddlers.

➤ *Bright and Early Books for Beginning Beginners* and *Beginner Books* (New York: Random House, Inc.); these two series are great fun for little ones; they tweak their senses of humor and age well. Look for the Dr. Seuss Cat in the Hat emblem on the spine.

➤ *Brown Bear, Brown Bear, What Do You See?* by Bill Martin, Jr., and John Archambault, illustrated by Eric Carle (New York: Henry Holt and Co., 1983); an introduction to colors through beautifully illustrated animals and repetitive text.

We all came from book-loving families and are book lovers ourselves, sharing a special fondness for classics from our own childhoods such as:

➤ H. A. Rey's _Curious George_

➤ A. A. Milne's _Winnie the Pooh_

➤ Ludwig Bemelman's _Madeline_

➤ Munro Leaf's _The Story of Ferdinand_

➤ Esphyr Sobodkina's _Caps for Sale_

➤ Laurent de Brunhoff's _Babar_ (although we worried about how our kids would take Babar's mother being killed off)

➤ Beatrix Potter's _Tales of Peter Rabbit_

➤ Watty Piper's recently reprinted _The Little Engine That Could_

➤ Maurice Sendak's _Where the Wild Things Are_

Many happy returns . . . to you all.